RECENT ADVANCES IN ANAEROBIC BACTERIOLOGY

NEW PERSPECTIVES IN CLINICAL MICROBIOLOGY

Brumfitt W, ed Hamilton-Miller JMT, assist. ed: New perspectives in clinical microbiology.
1978. ISBN 90-247-2074-5

Tyrrell DAJ, ed: Aspects of slow and persistent virus infections. 1979.
ISBN 90-247-2281-0

Brumfitt W, Curcio L, Silvestri L, eds: Combined antimicrobial therapy. 1979.
ISBN 90-247-2280-2

van Furth R, ed: Developments in antibiotic treatment of respiratory infections. 1981.
ISBN 90-247-2493-7

van Furth R, ed: Evaluation and management of hospital infections. 1982.
ISBN 90-247-2754-5

Kuwahara S, Pierce NF, eds: Advances in research on cholera and related diarrheas 1.
1983. ISBN 0-89838-592-X

Ristic M, Ambroise-Thomas P, Kreier J, eds: Malaria and babesiosis: Research findings
and control measures. 1984. ISBN 0-89838-675-6

Kuwahara S, Pierce NF, eds: Advances in research on cholera and related diarrheas 2.
1984. ISBN 0-89838-680-2

Takeda Y: Bacterial diarrheal diseases. 1984. ISBN 0-89838-681-0

Hill MJ, Borriello SP, Hardie JM, Hudson MJ, Lysons RJ, Tabaqchali S, eds: Models of
anaerobic infection.
1984. ISBN 0-89838-688-8

Taylor-Robinson D, ed: Clinical problems in sexually transmitted diseases.
1985. ISBN 0-89838-720-5

Borriello SP, Hardie JM, Drasar BS, Duerden BI, Hudson MJ, Lysons RJ, eds: Recent
advances in anaerobic bacteriology.
1987. ISBN 0-89838-847-3

RECENT ADVANCES IN ANAEROBIC BACTERIOLOGY

Proceedings of the fourth Anaerobic Discussion Group Symposium held at Churchill College, University of Cambridge, July 26–28, 1985

editors in chief:
S.P. BORRIELLO and J.M. HARDIE

editors:
B.S. DRASAR, B.I. DUERDEN, M.J. HUDSON and R.J. LYSONS

1987 **MARTINUS NIJHOFF PUBLISHERS**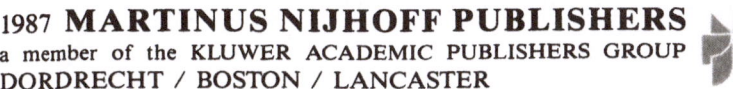
a member of the KLUWER ACADEMIC PUBLISHERS GROUP
DORDRECHT / BOSTON / LANCASTER

Distributors

for the United States and Canada: Kluwer Academic Publishers, P.O. Box 358, Accord Station, Hingham, MA 02018-0358, USA
for the UK and Ireland: Kluwer Academic Publishers, MTP Press Limited, Falcon House, Queen Square, Lancaster LA1 1RN, UK
for all other countries: Kluwer Academic Publishers Group, Distribution Center, P.O. Box 322, 3300 AH Dordrecht, The Netherlands

Library of Congress Cataloging in Publication Data

Anaerobe Discussion Group. Symposium (4th : 1985 :
   Churchill College)
   Recent advances in anaerobic bacteriology.

   (New perspectives in clinical microbiology ; 12)
   1. Bacteria, Anaerobic--Congresses. 2. Bacterial
diseases--Congresses. I. Borriello, S. Peter.
II. Hardie, J. M. III. Title. IV. Series. [DNLM:
1. Bacteria, Anaerobic--congresses. W3 AN533 4th 1985r /
QW 4 A532 1985r]
QR89.5.A23 1985   616.9'2   86-28482

ISBN 978-94-010-7978-5   ISBN 978-94-009-3293-7 (eBook)
DOI 10/1007/978-94-009-3293-7

Copyright

PREFACE

The Anaerobe Discussion Group (ADG) has organised four International Symposia, all at Churchill College, Cambridge. The first was held in July 1979, the second in July 1981, the third in July 1983, and this, the fourth, on July 26-28th, 1985. The proceedings of each of these meetings have been published (see below).

As on previous occasions, the scientific programme was designed to appeal to the wide range of interests represented by ADG members. The meeting was attended by delegates from all over the world, including medical micro-biologists, veterinarians, dentists, biochemists, geneticists and scientists from several other disciplines, all of whom share a common interest in anaerobic micro-organisms. The interchange of scientific information and ideas between the delegates in such pleasant surroundings was, as always, a valuable and rewarding experience.

Unlike previous Biennial Symposia in the series, this meeting was sponsored by a number of companies rather than by a single sponsor. Despite some intitial concern by the organising committee, this arrangement worked well and we are extremely grateful to all the companies who supported the meeting so generously. The names of the sponsors are listed individually in the acknowledgements section. We were also very pleased to welcome those companies who took part in the Trade Show during the meeting.

This book contains the papers given by invited contributors, followed by abstracts of the poster demonstration presented at the meeting.

S.P. Borriello
J.M. Hardie

List of Published Proceedings of Previous ADG Symposia

1. Pathogenic, Immunological and Therapeutic Aspects of
    Anaerobic Infections. Edited by J.G. Collee and S.
    Tabaqchali. Research and Clinical Forums 1, No.3.
    (1979)

2. Control of the Alimentary Flora in Health and
    Disease. Edited by S. Tabaqchali and the Steering
    Committee of the Anaerobe Discussion Group, The
    European Journal of Chemotherapy and Antibiotics 2,
    No. 1 (1982).

3. Models of Anaerobic Infection. Edited by M.J.Hill and
    the Steering Committee of Anaerobe Discussion Group.
    Martinus Nijhoff (1984) ISBN 0-89838-688-8.

CONTENTS

Preface V

Acknowledgements and List of Sponsors XI

Photograph of the Organizing Committee XIII

Introduction to the Anaerobe Discussion Group Ltd. XV

List of Contributors XVII

Section 1. Dealing with Anaerobes

Coping with anaerobes in a routine laboratory.
W.A.Hyde. 3

Enzyme profiles as an aid to the identification of anaerobes.
M.W.D. Wren and Josephine M. Silles. 17

Sensitivity testing and MIC determination of obligate anaerobes.
D. Felmingham 28

Section 2. Anaerobes and Gastrointestinal Disease

Clostridium perfringens enterotoxin-associated diarrhoea.
S.P. Borriello, H.E. Larson, Fiona E. Barclay and A.R. Welch. 33

Gastrointestinal *Campylobacter*-like organisms.
Jean M. Dolby. 43

Intestinal spirochetosis in man and other animals.
Kari Hovind-Hougen. 56

Anaerobes and inflammatory bowel disease.
M.J. Hudson. 60

Section 3. Antibiotics and Anaerobes

Newer antibiotics active againsts *Bacteriodes fragilis*: comparison with older agents.
A. Eley and D. Greenwood. 75

Interaction of antibiotics, anaerobic bacteria and host defences.
C.G. Gemmell. 90

Antibiotics, anaerobes and colonization resistance.
D. van der Waaij. 100

Antibiotic manipulation of the rumen microflora. The effects of avoparcin and monensin on the relase of tritium from labelled cellulose by *Bacteroides succinogenes* and the rumen fungus *Neocallimastic frontalis*.
C.S. Stewart, Sylvia H. Duncan and K.N. Joblin. 108

Section 4. Advances in Genetic Manipulation and the
Commercial Exploitation of Anaerobes

Genetic approaches with methanogens important in
mesophilic anaerobic digestion.
Jane E. Harris, D.M. Evans, Margaret R. Knox and D.B.
Archer.   123

Genetic analysis of toxin determinants of *Clostridium
perfringens*.
N.F. Fairweather, D.J. Pickard, D.M. Morrissey, Valerie A.
Lyness and G. Dougan.   138

Sulphate reducing bacteria and the offshore oil industry.
W.A. Hamilton.   148

Prospects for the genetic manipulation of rumen
microorganisms.
G.P. Hazlewood, S.P. Mann, C.G. Orpin and M.P.M. Romanick.   162

Commercial exploitation of cellulolytic anaerobes.
R. Sleat.   177

Section 5. Anaerobes and Genital Tract Infections

The anaerobic bacterial flora of the vagina in health and
disease.
M. Wilks and Soad Tabaqchali.   195

Mobiluncus and bacterial vaginosis.
Ada Vetere, S.P. Borriello and D. Taylor-Robinson.   205

Differentiation of *Mobiluncus* species by pyrolysis gas-
liquid chromatography.
T.G. Winstanley, J.M. Hindmarch and J.T. Magee.   215

Anaerobes in non-gonococcal urethritis, balanoposthitis and
genital ulcers.
B.I. Duerden.   231

Section 6. Taxonomy of Anaerobes

Anaerobic Archaebacteria.
W.D. Grant.   245

Recent advances in the taxonomy of the genus *Bacteroides*.
M.D. Collins and H.N. Shah.   249

The taxonomy of the asaccharolytic anaerobic Gram-
positive cocci.
Elizabeth A. Taylor and I. Phillips.   259

Taxonomy of spiral and curved clostridia.
R.J. Carman, Elizabeth P. Cato and T.D. Wilkins.   271

Abstracts of posters presented at the Fourth Anaerobe
Discussion Group Biennial Symposium, 1985.   281

ACKNOWLEDGEMENTS AND LIST OF SPONSORS

The ADG committee are most grateful to Ms. Nina Liu for all her help with the organization of the 4th Biennial Symposium, and to Miss A.E. Hammerton and her staff at Churchill College, cambridge, for the excellent local arrangements.

We are pleased to acknowledge the assistance received from the University of London Computer Centre, particularly Clare Steward and John Gilbert, and from Bob Nash and Jenny Wale at the London Hospital Medical College, during the preparation and editing of these proceedings.

No meeting of this kind can be organised without adequate financial support and we are extremely grateful to the following companies for their generous sponsorship:

    Don Whitely Scientific Ltd.
    May and Baker Ltd.
    Stuart Pharmaceuticals Ltd./ICI p.l.c.
    Upjohn Ltd.
    Coralab Research
    Pfizer Ltd.
    Searle Research and Development
    Cooper's Animal Health
    Merck Sharp and Dohme Ltd.
    Wellcome Biotechnology

In addition to these companies, bursaries to enable selected younger workers to attend the meeting were kindly provided by:

    Abbott Laboratories Ltd.,
    Oxoid Ltd.
    E.R. Squibb and Sons Ltd.
    Janssen Pharmaceuticals Ltd
    The Anaerobe Discussion Group Ltd.

Photographs were taken by Mr. Phillip J. Reed, (Clinical Research Centre, Watford Road, Harrow, Middlesex HA1 3UJ).

ANAEROBE DISCUSSION GROUP

4th Biennial Symposium, Churchill College, Cambridge

26th – 28th July, 1986

ORGANIZING COMMITTEE

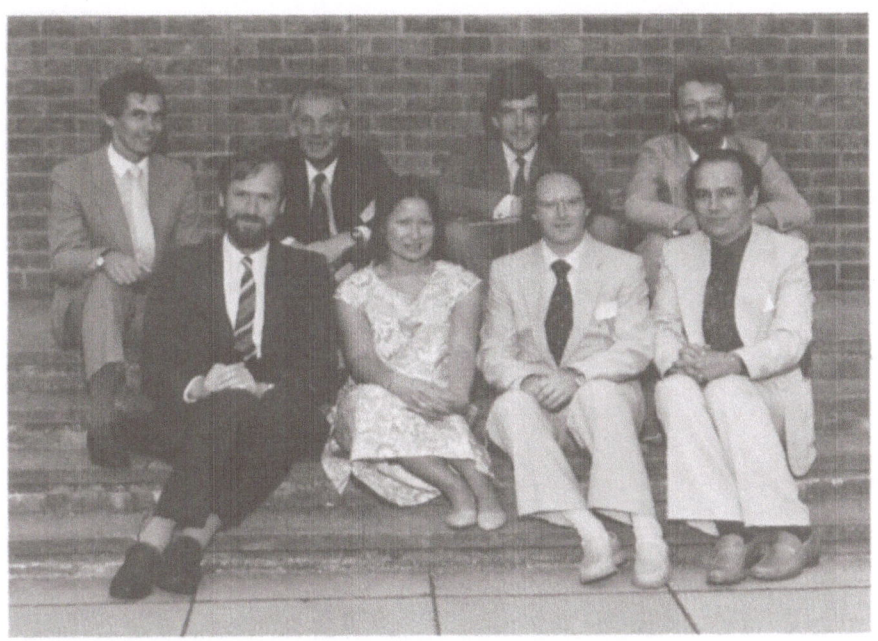

From left to right:
Back row
    David Jackson,   Brian Capel,   Michael   Hudson,   Peter
    Borriello

Front row
    Jeremy Hardie, Nina Liu, Brian Duerden, Bo Drasar

    (absent from photograph, Dick Lysons)

INTRODUCTION TO THE ANAEROBE DISCUSSION GROUP

The Anaerobe Discussion Group (ADG) was formed in 1975 when 16 people working on various aspects of anaerobe bacteriology met at the Central Public Health Laboratory, London, to exchange information and ideas. The intial group included people interested in human infection, the human gut, dental bacteriology, veterinary bacteriology and toxicology and it quickly became apparent that the various subgroups could benefit greatly from each other's expertise, so we have attempted to maintain this mix of interests and, where possible, to extend it. The aim of this group is to raise the technical standards of anaerobic bacteriology to the maximum and to increase the general awareness of the function of anaerobic bacteria in health and disease, and in the environment. It holds three or four meetings a year, usually on Tuesday afternoons in or around London, although a few "country" meetings have been held further afield in recent years. Wherever possible, younger workers are encouraged to present their research findings at these half-day meetings.

Until recently the ADG had no formal constitution, but in 1985 a constitution was adopted and the group became the ADG Ltd. Over 250 names are on the mailing list and average attendance at the regular meetings during recent years has been around 60-70. Although many of the members are in the London area, an increasing number come from more distant parts of the country and abroad. The Biennial Symposia at Cambridge have always been particularly well attended (over 200 delegates in 1985) and have attracted contributors from many countries around the world.

The ADG is run by a committee, currently consisting of Jeremy Hardie (Chairman; London Hospital Medical College), Brian Capel (Treasurer; CAMR), Michael Hudson (CAMR), Brian Duerden (University of Sheffield Medical School), Richard Lysons (ARC, Compton), Bo Drasar (London School of Hygiene and Tropical Medicine), Peter Borriello (Clinical Research Centre, Northwick Park Hospital) and David Jackson (May and Baker Ltd.).

The group especially welcomes people who are new to the field of anaerobic bacteriology, whatever their scientific background, and anyone interested in joining should contact one of the committee members. Presently, the membership fee is £3:00 p.a. for UK residents and £4:00 pa for overseas members. Fees may be paid in advance for periods of one or three years.

J.M. Hardie

LIST OF CONTRIBUTORS

Archer, D.B.	AFRC Food Research Institute – Norwich, Colney Lane, Norwich NR4 7UA
Barclay, Fiona E.	Division of Communicable Diseases, Clinical Research Centre, Watford Road, Harrow, Middlesex HA1 3UJ
Borriello, S.P.	" " "
Carman, R.J.	Department of Anaerobic Microbiology, Virginia Polytechnic Institute and State University ,Blacksburg, Virginia 24061, U.S.A.
Cato, Elizabeth P.	" " "
Collins, M.D.	Department of Food Microbiology, Food Research Institute, Shinfield, Reading RG2 9AT
Dolby, Jean M.	Division of Communicable Diseases, Clinical Research Centre, Watford Road, Harrow, Middlesex HA1 3UJ
Dougan, G.	Bacterial Genetics Group, Department of Molecular Biology, Wellcome Biotechnology Ltd., Beckenham, Kent
Duerden, B.I.	Department of Medical Microbiology, University of Sheffield Medical School, Beech Hill Road, Sheffield S10 2RX
Duncan, Sylvia H.	Rowett Research Insitute, Bucksburn, Aberdeen AB2 9SB
Eley, A.	Department of Microbiology and PHLS Laboratory, University Hospital, Queen's Medical Centre, Nottingham NG7 7UH
Evans, D.M.	AFRC Food Research Institute Norwich, Colney Lane, Norwich NR4 7UA
Fairweather, N.F.	Bacterial Genetics Group, Department of Molecular Biology, Wellcome Biotechnology, Beckenham, Kent
Felmingham, D.	Clinical Microbiology, University College Hospital, Grafton Way, London WC1E 6AU
Gemmel, C.G.	Department of Bacteriology, University of Glasgow Medical School, Royal Infirmary, Glasgow
Greenwood, D.	Department of Microbiology and PHLS Laboratory, University Hospital, Queen's Medical Centre, Nottingham, NG7 2UH

Hamilton,W.A.   Department of Microbiology, Marischal
                       College, University of Aberdeen,
                       Aberdeen AB9 1AS

Hardie, J.M.   Department of Oral Microbiology, The
                       London Hospital Medical College,
                       Turner Street, London E1 2AD

Harris, Jane E.   AFRC Food Research Institute -
                       Norwich, Colney Lane, Norwich NR4 7UA

Hazelwood, G.P.   Department of Biochemistry, AFRC
                       Institute of Animal Physiology,
                       Babraham, Cambridge CB2 4AT

Hindmarch, J.M.   Department of Bacteriology, Royal
                       Hallamshire Hospital, Sheffield S10
                       2JF

Hovind-Hougen, Kari   State Veterinary Serum Laboratory,
                       Copenhagen, Denmark

Hudson, M.J.   Bacterial Metabolism Research
                       Laboratory, PHLS Centre for Applied
                       Microbiology and Research, Porton Down,
                       Salisbury, Wilts. SP4 0JG

Hyde, W.A.   Company Microbiologist, Lab M. Ltd.

Joblin, K.N.   DSIR, Palmerston North, New Zealand

Knox, Margaret R.   AFRC Food Research Institute -
                       Norwich, Colney Lane, Norwich NR4 7UA

Larson, H.E.   Division of Communicable Diseases,
                       Clinical Research Centre, Watford
                       Road, Harrow, Middlesex HA1 3UJ

Lyness, Valerie A.   Bacterial Genetics Group, Department
                       of Molecular Biology, Wellcome
                       Biotechnology Ltd., Beckenham, Kent

Magee, J.T.   Department of Bacteriology,
                       Children's Hospital, Western Bank,
                       Sheffield S10 2TH

Mann, S.P.   AFRC Institute of Animal Physiology,
                       Babraham, Cambridge CB2 4AT

Morrissey, P.M.   Bacterial Genetics Group, Department
                       of Molecular Biology, Wellcome
                       Biotechnology Ltd., Beckenham, Kent

Orpin, C.G.   AFRC Institute of Animal Physiology,
                       Babraham, Cambridge CB2 4AT

Phillips, I.   Department of Medical Microbiology,
                       St. Thomas' Hospital, London SE1

Pickard, D.J.   Bacterial Genetics Group, Department
                       of Molecular Biology, Wellcome
                       Biotechnology Ltd., Beckenham, Kent

Hamilton,W.A.   Department of Microbiology, Marischal
                         College, University of Aberdeen,
                         Aberdeen AB9 1AS

Hardie, J.M.   Department of Oral Microbiology, The
                         London Hospital Medical College,
                         Turner Street, London E1 2AD

Harris, Jane E.   AFRC Food Research Institute –
                         Norwich, Colney Lane, Norwich NR4 7UA

Hazelwood, G.P.   Department of Biochemistry, AFRC
                         Institute of Animal Physiology,
                         Babraham, Cambridge CB2 4AT

Hindmarch, J.M.   Department of Bacteriology, Royal
                         Hallamshire Hospital, Sheffield S10
                         2JF

Hovind-Hougen, Kari   State Veterinary Serum Laboratory,
                         Copenhagen, Denmark

Hudson, M.J.   Bacterial Metabolism Research
                         Laboratory, PHLS Centre for Applied Microbiolog
                         and Research, Porton Down, Salisbury,
                         Wilts. SP4 0JG

Hyde, W.A.   Company Microbiologist, Lab M. Ltd.

Joblin, K.N.   DSIR, Palmerston North, New Zealand

Knox, Margaret R.   AFRC Food Research Institute –
                         Norwich, Colney Lane, Norwich NR4 7UA

Larson, H.E.   Division of Communicable Diseases,
                         Clinical Research Centre, Watford
                         Road, Harrow, Middlesex HA1 3UJ

Lyness, Valerie A.   Bacterial Genetics Group, Department
                         of Molecular Biology, Wellcome
                         Biotechnology Ltd., Beckenham, Kent

Magee, J.T.   Department of Bacteriology,
                         Children's Hospital, Western Bank,
                         Sheffield S10 2TH

Mann, S.P.   AFRC Institute of Animal Physiology,
                         Babraham, Cambridge CB2 4AT

Morrissey, P.M.   Bacterial Genetics Group, Department
                         of Molecular Biology, Wellcome
                         Biotechnology Ltd., Beckenham, Kent

Orpin, C.G.   AFRC Institute of Animal Physiology,
                         Babraham, Cambridge CB2 4AT

Phillips, I.   Department of Medical Microbiology,
                         St. Thomas' Hospital, London SE1

Pickard, D.J.   Bacterial Genetics Group, Department
                         of Molecular Biology, Wellcome
                         Biotechnology Ltd., Beckenham, Kent

Romaniec, M.P.M.	AFRC Institute of Animal Physiology, Babraham, Cambridge CB2 4AT
Shah, H.,N.	Department of Oral Microbiology, The London Hospital Medical College, Turner Street, London E1 2AD
Silles, Josephine M.	Department of Pathology, North Middlesex Hospital, Silver Street, Edmonton, London N18
Sleat, R.	Biotechnica Ltd., 5 Chiltern Close, Llanishen, Cardiff CF4 5DL
Stewart, C.S.	Rowett Research Institute, Bucksburn, Aberdeen, AB2 9SB
Tabaqchali, Soad	Department of Medical Microbiology, St. Bartholomew's Hospital Medical College, West Smithfield, London EC1A 7BE
Taylor,Elizabeth A.	Merck, Sharp and Dohme, Hertford Road, Hoddesdon, Hertfordshire
Taylor-Robinson,D.	Division of Sexually Transmitted Diseases, Clinical Research Centre, Watford Road, Harrow, Middlesex HA1 3UJ
Van der Waaij, D.	Laboratory for Medical Microbiology, University of Groningen, The Netherlands
Vetere, Ada	Division of Sexually Transmitted Diseases, Clinical Research Centre, Watford Road, Harrow, Middlesex HA1 3UJ
Welch, A.R.	Divison of Communicable Diseases, Clinical Research Centre, Watford Road, Harrow, Middlesex HA1 3UJ
Wilkins, T.D.	Department of Anaerobic Microbiology, Virginia Polytechnic Institute and State University, Blacksburg, Virginia 24061, U.S.A.
Wilks, M.	Department of Medical Microbiology, St. Bartholomew's Hospital Medical College, West Smithfield, London EC1A 7BE
Winstanley, T.	Department of Bacteriology, Royal Hallamshire Hospital, Sheffield S10 2JF
Wren, M.W.D.	Department of Pathology, North Middlesex Hospital, Silver Street, Edmonton, London N18

SECTION 1.   DEALING WITH ANAEROBES

Chairman of Session : Professor J.G. Collee

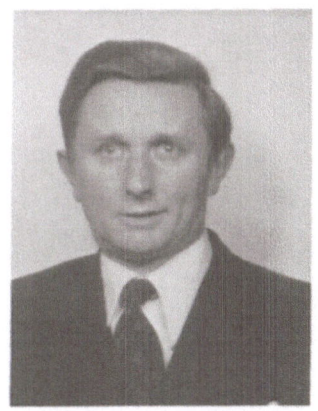

Professor J.G. Collee

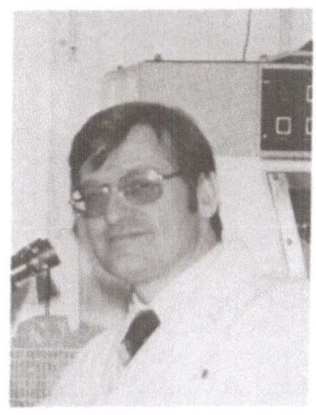

W.A. Hyde

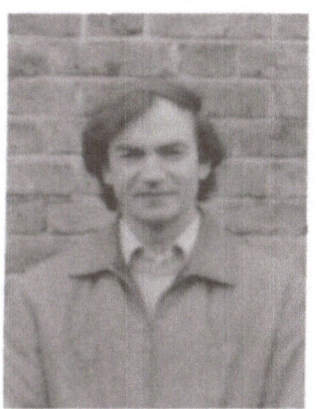

M.W.D. Wren

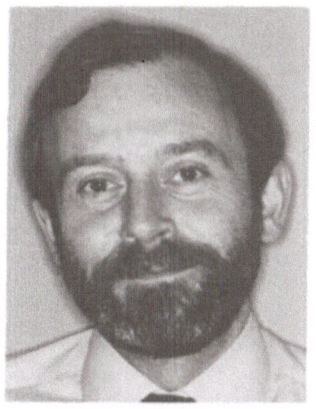

D. Felmingham

CHAPTER 1

COPING WITH ANAEROBES IN A ROUTINE HOSPITAL LABORATORY

W. A. Hyde,

Company Microbiologist, LAB M Ltd.,
(Previously S.C.M.L.S.O. Salford Health Authority)

Contents

Introduction

Coping with anaerobes

    swabs

    sputa

    blood cultures

    pus

Plating out

    media

Incubation

    anaerobic Cabinets

    examination at 48 hrs.

    picking off

Identification

Remaining problems

References

INTRODUCTION

Few laboratories can cope well with anaerobes. Those which can do so by educating in the effective collection and transport of samples, and emphasis is placed on acquiring samples of pus whenever possible in preference to swabs. If swabs must be used they should be collected in anaerobic transport medium and kept at 4°C. until inoculation.

Sputum samples are only useful for gas liquid chromato-graphy (G.L.C.) culture is usually not worthwhile because of oral contamination, which can be avoided by samples taken at bronchoscopy. When culturing of anaerobes from blood a rich anaerobic medium is required; polymicrobial septicaemia with mixtures of aerobes and anaerobes can sometimes occur - but selective media for sub-culture - or direct G.L.C. on the broth will quickly detect these mixtures. *Propionibacterium acnes* in blood cultures can be mistaken for actinomyces species, because of a tendency to branch in young cultures.

Samples of pus need the same urgent treatment as that given to cerebro-spinal fluid (C.S.F.). Rapid tests on the sample including Gram Stain, direct fluorescence and G.L.C. will detect the majority of anaerobe infections, but information from Gram films should be used cautiously.

Plating can be done on the open bench, but a transfer jar is recommended to prevent loss of viability. Selective media is essential to separate mixed cultures and these should be incubated in an anaerobic incubator.

The organisation of work around the cabinet needs

special worksheets and careful selection and organisational procedures.

Picking-off of isolates is done on the open bench
using a stereo microscope and a straight wire. Identification of these isolates can be carried out with either
Minitek or API 20 A - or an "in house" system. Identification sensitivity discs together with other identification tests in tablet form can be used. New methods of
enzyme identification are also available.

The need for more information regarding pathogenic
significance of species and mixtures - and their rapid
identification is emphasised.

COPING WITH ANAEROBES

The majority of routine hospital laboratories cannot
isolate and identify anaerobes with the same facility as
aerobes. There are many causes for this discrepancy, but
the main one is associated with the rapid expansion of our
awareness of anaerobes following the introduction of
better methods of isolation, the introduction of the
Gaspak, (B.B.L. Ltd.) and the publication of the anaerobe
manual of the Virginia Polytechnic Institute (1) in the
early 1970's. Unfortunately, this increase in isolation
and the expanded taxonomy was not accompanied by an
increase in our knowledge regarding which of the new
species had pathogenic significance.

Table 1.   Taxonomy of Anaerobes in Many Routine Laboratories 1970

Gram Negative Rods	–	*Bacteroides*
Gram Positive Cocci	–	*Anaerobic Streptococci*
Gram Negative Cocci	–	*Veillonella*
Gram Positive Sporing Bacilli	–	*Clostridium welchii*
		Clostridium tetanii
		Clostridium sp.
Gram Positive Non-sporing Bacilli	–	*Anaerobic diphtheroids*

The taxonomy used by many clinical laboratories in the early seventies was fairly rudimentary and many laboratories reported their anaerobe isolates as shown in table 1.

Faced with these new genera many microbiologists asked:

How do we collect and transport samples to isolate these bacteria?
How do we grow, and identify them?
How do we ascertain their sensitivity to antibiotics?
How do we know which are significant when asked?

and last but of considerable importance – how can we afford all this new work? – often with no increase in budget allowance. Some microbiologists came to the conclusion they could not cope with these problems and resorted to simply reporting "Anaerobes present sensitive to metronidazole".

Those who decided to tackle the isolation and identification of anaerobes first approached their colleagues in the medical and nursing professions to make them aware of the new situation and seek help in ensuring that good specimens were taken and transported to the laboratory without delay. They were shown the benefits obtained with collection of pus wherever possible, and when it became necessary to take swabs, the importance of trying to get an expressed sample – which would more likely reflect the situation deeper in the wound.

Swabs. There are many problems associated with collection of swabs; not least the finding by Collee (2) that only 3 –5% of bacteria which are taken onto the swab are released onto the culture plate. The same paper, and subsequent work, has shown that anaerobes die on dry swabs quickly, but Hill (3) showed that they can be maintained in a viable state by the use of a suitable transport medium. Ashurst (4) also found that if swabs in transport media are kept at +4°C anaerobes maintained their viability much longer than at 20°C.

Sputa. Sputum samples from a patient suffering from an anaerobic lung infection are often composed of thin smelly pus, but smell can be absent, as in infections caused by members of the *Fusobacterium* genus, or misleading when present in an infection caused by *Proteus* sp.

Routine culture of sputum for anaerobes is not a worthwhile procedure because of the contamination of the sputum with large numbers of anaerobic bacteria from the oral cavity, and, as previously stated, we do not as yet have a clear picture of the pathogenic properties of the varying mixtures of anaerobes often present in the upper respiratory tract flora found in lung infections. There is rarely a single organism involved in anaerobe infections – unlike most aerobic infections. Trans- tracheal aspirate is a method advocated by Finegold (5), a procedure which has found little favour in this country, but samples taken during bronchoscopy can prove useful in culturing anaerobes from lung infections.

The most valuable technique available in diagnosing anaerobic lung infections is analysis of the sputum by G.L.C. This technique detects the presence of volatile fatty acids, acetic and propionic acids are often found in aerobic infections but longer chain acids such as N-butyric are only produced by anaerobic bacteria, and the presence of these acids is diagnostic of an anaerobe infection. They are not found in sputum from patients suffering from aerobic infections in spite of anaerobe bacterial contamination of the sputum from the upper respiratory tract.

Blood cultures. The anaerobic culture medium must, of course, be rich and well reduced, capable of re-reducing itself after the cap has been removed to sample the broth - or there must be an anaerobic gas replacement system such as Bactec (Johnston Laboratories).

Mixed infections are sometimes missed, in the excitement of the discovery of *Escherichia coli* or *Streptococcus milleri* growing well on the aerobic plates and can lead to ignoring the presence of *Bacteroides fragilis* or *Peptostreptococcus anaerobius* on the anaerobic plates. This problem can be overcome using selective anaerobic plates, or a metronidazole disc on the inoculum of the anaerobe plate.

G.L.C. again can detect the mixture in most cases, and it can, sometimes, also give an indication of the type of aerobe present.

A common isolate from blood cultures which can cause confusion is *Proprionibacterium acnes*, which on primary isolation in young culture shows branching to such an extent that it has been confused with Actinomyces species. On ageing the cultures become more regular and much less branched, but, once more, G.L.C. analysis of broth will give a definite diagnosis.

Pus. If a pot of pus arrives in the laboratory, even unannounced, it should be treated with the same urgency as that given to a purulent C.S.F. If this is done routinely the rapid tests which can be carried out on the specimen can be reported that day, saving both invaluable time in the diagnosis for the patient, and improving the reputation of the laboratory.

These rapid tests are:

    1.   Gram-film
    2.   Direct autofluorescence detection
    3.   G.L.C.

Using these tests Phillips, Eykyn & Taylor (6) obtained the following results:

There can be difficulties of misdiagnosis using Gram-film alone. For example, *Bacillus cereus* is almost indistinguishable morphologically from *Clostridium perfringens*, and anaerobic, Gram positive cocci are impossible to differentiate from aerobic cocci.

On the other hand, positive G.L.C. result can give a definite diagnosis. If G.L.C. on pus is negative then it is probably unlikely that anaerobes are causing the infection.

Table 2. Efficiency of Combined Gram Stain, U.V. Fluorescence, and Direct G.L.C. in the Diagnosis of Anaerobic Infection in 112 Samples of Pus.

Gram	Fluorescence	G.L.C.	Percent
+	+	+	55
+	−	+	31
−	−	+	7
+	−	−	4
−	−	−	4

Direct salmon pink fluorescence is usually indicative of the presence of one of the melaninogenicus group of anaerobes, but it must be remembered that *Corynebacterium minutissimum* can also produce similar fluorescence.

PLATING OUT

This can be carried out on the open bench so long as there is not a long delay before enough plates are accumulated to fill a jar, or transfer chamber of a cabinet. This can be overcome by the use of a transfer jar continuously flushed with CO_2 . This was suggested by Ellner in the early 1970's (7). An updated modification of this could be made by substitution of the large Whitley jar with its valve cores removed and connected to CO_2 source. Media. Wren's (8) suggestions for isolation media are still generally sound, and table 3 should prove instructive.

Pre-reduced plates are unnecessary, but fresh plates, eg. less than 24 hrs. old, should be used.

The modification which I would suggest is the use of a base medium such as Wilkens-Chalgren (Oxoid) or Fastidious Anaerobe Agar (Lab M). The cost of large numbers of selective plates can be overcome by the use of segmented plates with a different medium in each segment.

Table 3.

MEDIA	
Blood agar + Vit. K + Haemin	– Most Significant Anaerobes
Blood agar + Vit. K + Haemin + Nalidixic acid + Tween	– *Fusobacterium, Melaninogenicus* group, Cocci.
Blood agar + Neomycin	– *Clostridium, fragilis* group, some cocci
Blood agar + Vit. K + Haemin + Brilliant Green + Rifampicin	– *Fusobacterium*
Willis & Hobbs	– *Clostridium*

INCUBATION

Anaerobic jars plus either Gaspak (B.B.L. Ltd,) or Gaskit (Oxoid) are not an economically sound proposition for the larger laboratory when compared to the economics of buying and running an anaerobe cabinet. This is even more true now with the advent of a new cabinet (9) which does not need the special gas mixture (80% Nitrogen 10% carbon dioxide and 10% hydrogen), but uses valves to mix the gas in the chamber. Jars are still useful for such specimens of throat swab for haemolytic streptococci and sputum for pneumococci, and also for when the cabinet breaks down! The most telling argument against jars must be the logistical problem of duplicating plates and jars to be examined at 24 and 48 hrs., and the picking of colonies from large numbers of aerobe and anaerobic plates - before the anaerobic plates can be returned, to the jar, the loss of anaerobes must be enormous.

Anaerobic cabinets. The separation of reading and recording of the anaerobic and aerobic plates when an anaerobic cabinet is introduced into the laboratory poses organisational difficulties. To help overcome these problems, the laboratory at Oldham D.G.H. introduced a work-sheet, Table 4.

Table 4. Laboratory Worksheet.

Day	Date				
Lab.No.	Name	Ward	Clinical Details	Aerobes Growth	Anaerobes Identify

This is initially filled in by the staff dealing with the sample and a red metal flag (10) is attached to all forms from specimens incubated in the anaerobe cabinet. The staffing of the bench which reads the plates from pus and swabs etc. is separated into aerobic and anaerobic sections, jointly under the control of a senior or chief M.L.S.O.

Examination of plates at 24 hrs.   Only brief details of the aerobic growth are entered on the form eg. "Staphs", "Strepts", "coliform", "diphtheroids" etc. just to give the anaerobe section some idea of which facultative organisms could be expected.

Table 5. Workflow Pus Bench 24 hours

Aerobe Section	Anaerobe Section
Reads Aerobic & CO_2	Reads Anaerobic Plates
Re-incubates & Sub-cultures	Picks significant growths
"No Growth"	Re-incubate all plates
Writes Aerobic Report onto Worksheet	

The only plate to be removed from the cabinet at this time should be the neomycin blood agar, which shows evidence of *Clostridia* or *Bacteroides* species. The others must be left in, or picked off in the cabinet, otherwise serious loss of vulnerable micro-colonies would result (11).

Examination at 48 hrs. This is decision time. Which specimens have grown anaerobes? Which are worth identifying? Which plates need re-incubating, are there any anaerobes on the "No Growth" aerobic specimens? Before identifying, it is always worth a member of the medical staff ringing the ward to assess the nature of the lesion and the condition of the patient. To try to attempt to identify all anaerobes isolated is expensive, unnecessary and unrealistic.

PICKING-OFF

After 48 hrs. incubation colony picks can be performed on the open bench. It is easier to use a plate microscope on the open bench, and picking-off using this microscope

is essential if pure growth are to be obtained. The
"pick-offs" can be transferred to 1/4 or 1/6 plates to be
incubated in CO_2 and anaerobically. These pure growths
can then be used to inoculate other identification media.

IDENTIFICATION

The first difficulty the anaerobic bacteriologist faces
is: Is this organism Gram-negative or is it Gram-positive
pretending to be Gram-negative?

This can be clarified by the technique suggested by
Gregersen in 1978 (12). This test consists of rubbing a
colony onto a drop of 3% KOH on a slide. If the organism is
Gram-negative the emulsion can be drawn up with a wire loop as
stringy mucus.

Table 6. Workflow Pus Bench 48 hrs.

Aerobe Section	Anaerobe Section
Reads all aerobic plates & reports growth	Reads 48 hr. growths
Passes "No Growth" reports to Anaerobe Section	Assesses which need processing
Passes Red Flag Forms to Anaerobe Section	Checks all aerobe "No Growth" Reports
	Adds preliminary anaerobe reports to forms with Red Flags
	Re-incubates for 3 more days plates ? Anaerobic infections.

Sutter and Finegold (13) in 1971 introduced high
strength antibiotic discs as part of a system to help
identify anaerobes. These discs are still useful, but are
often used alone, in which case the results can be misleading. The other tests which they suggested were Gram

stain, egg yolk reaction, bile sensitivity and aesculin
hydrolysis.

These are useful and easy tests and the latter two
can be performed using commercially available substrate
tablets.

Carbohydrate fermentations are an essential feature
of anaerobe identification. With clostridia, the old
technique of the red hot nail into peptone water sugars is
still of value, but this method has been superseded by "In
house" and commercial systems of identification.

The most popular of the commercial methods are API 20A
(API Ltd.) and Minitek (B.B.L. Ltd.). API 20A was introduced in 1974. In practice it is sometimes difficult to
read and its data base used to be inadequate. However,
good results can be obtained if strict attention is paid
to manufacturer's instruction. Minitek was introduced In
1980, it is apparently easier to read than API 20 A and
its data manual is extensive and has much valuable information, especially on supplementary tests, including
G.L.C.

In comparisons of both systems, experienced workers
have found little difference between the results obtained.

One of the most useful, and perhaps simple, fermentation techniques is that introduced by Ken Phillips at
the Luton Anaerobe Reference Laboratory(14). This consists
of the use of a carbohydrate free blood agar plate whIch
is flooded with concentrated sterile sugar solution and
allowed to dry. The organisms to be tested are inoculated
onto sections of the plate. When an organism ferments the
sugar haemolysis often results. To confirm fermentation,a
plug of the medium is removed and a drop of indicator is
applied. Positive and negative controls can be used on

the same plates. This method is still in use at Luton. It has been shown that G.L.C. can also be carried out on plugs of agar removed from under colonies, even on primary plates of *C.difficile* (15).

Recent advances in identification are now showing the value of rapid enzyme tests on anaerobe isolates. These can be carried out using home-made reagents (16), using API ZYM (API Ltd) or Rosco tablets (Rosco Diagnostica, Denmark).

REMAINING PROBLEMS

There are problems which a routine clinical laboratory have still only partially answered. The identification systems are being made easier, but what the routine clinical laboratory needs in order to cope with anaerobes is information on which are the pathogens we should be looking for, and a short range of simple, speedy, tests to identify them.

References

1   Holdeman, L.V., Moore, W.E.C. (ed) 1972. Anaerobe
     Laboratory Manual 2nd ed. Virginia Polytechnic
     Institute, Blacksburg.

2   Collee, J.G., Watt, B., Brown R., Johnstone, S. 1973.
     The Recovery of Anaerobic Bacteria from Swabs.
     J. Hyg., Camb. 72: 339.

3   Hill, G., 1978. Effects of Storage in an Anaerobic
     Transport System on Bacteria in Known Polymicrobial
     Mixtures and in Clinical Specimens.
     J. Clin. Microbiol. 6: 680 - 688.

4   Ashurst, A. Leighton Hospital, Personal Communication

5   Finegold. S.M. 1977. Anaerobic Bacteria in Human
     Disease. Academic Press, New York.

6   Phillips, I., Eykyn, S., Taylor, E. 1980. The Rapid
     Laboratory Diagnosis of Anaerobic Infection.
     Infection: 8 (Suppl.2): 155 - 158.

7   Ellner, P.D., Granato, P.A., May, C.B., 1973.
     Recovery and Identification of Anaerobes: A System
     Suitable for the Routine Clinical Laboratory.
     Appl. Micro. 6: 904-913.

8   Wren, M.W.D. 1980. Multiple Selective Media for
     Isolation of Anaerobic Bacteria from Clinical
     Specimens. J. Clin. Pathol. 33: 61 - 65.

9   Whitley, Anaerobic Cabinet Mk. 111. Don. Whitley
     Scientific Ltd., Shipley, West Yorkshire.

10   SHUNIC SIGNALS, Gunnells Wood Road, Stevenage.

11   Wren, M.W.D. 1977. Cultivation of Clinical Specimens
     for Anaerobic Bacteria: Bacteriological Comparison
     of Specimens. J. Med. Microbiol. 10: 195 - 201.

12   Gregersen, T., 1978. Rapid Method for Distinction of
     Gram Negative from Gram Positive Bacteria.
     Eur. J. Appl. Microbiol. Biotechnol. 5: 123 - 127.

13   Sutter, V.L., Finegold, S.M., 1971. Antibiotic Disc
     susceptibility Tests for Rapid Presumptive
     Identification of Gram Negative Anaerobic Bacilli.
     Appl. Microbiol. 1: 13 - 20.

14   Phillips, K.D., 1976. A Simple and Sensitive
     Technique for Determining the Fermentation Reactions
     of Non-sporing Anaerobes.
     J. Appl. Bacteriol. 41: 325 - 328.

15   Makin, T., 1984. Rapid Identification of *Clostridium
     difficile* by Direct Detection of Volatile Organic
     Acids From Primary Isolation Media.
     J. Clin. Pathol. 37 : 711-712.

16   Wren, M.W.D. 1985. Proceedings of 4th Biennial
     Meeting of the Anaerobe Discussion Group.

CHAPTER 2

ENZYME PROFILES AS AN AID IN THE IDENTIFICATION OF ANAEROBES

M.W.D. Wren & Josephine M. Silles

North Middlsex Hospital, Silver Street, Edmonton, London, N1B 1QK.

Contents

Introduction

Materials and Methods

Results

      Nagler positive clostridia

      Nagler negative clostridia

      The *Bacteroidaceae*

      The anaerobic cocci

Discussion

References

INTRODUCTION

The basis of identifying clinically important anaerobic bacteria has traditionally relied on the use of sugar fermentation, together with other tests such as indole, aesculin hydrolysis, nitrate reduction and growth characteristics (e.g. growth in the presence of bile) coupled with gas liquid chromatography (GLC) of metabolic end products of fermentation (1,2). However, a good number of anaerobes of clinical interest are either asaccharolytic (e.g. the anaerobic cocci) or, are difficult to separate, such as some of the fusobacteria. Moreover, the time taken to incubate and read such tests may mean that several days are necessary to reach a final identification.

Clearly any method which can reduce the time taken to reach an answer would benefit both the patient and the clinician. The use of preformed enzymes as an aid in the identification of anaerobic bacteria can achieve these aims for two reasons. Firstly identification can be achieved in a much shorter time (i.e. 4 hrs). Secondly it may be possible to achieve a more accurate identification particularly with asaccharolytic strains where many of the traditional tests are repeatedly negative.

The techniques of rapid enzyme identification of bacteria are not new and early attempts have shown some success with the Bacillus genus(3), the Enterobacteriaceae (4), Actinomyces (5) and some anaerobic Gram-negative rods (6).

This paper presents the results obtained when testing for two major groups of enzymes, the carbohydrate glycosidases and the amino acid arylamidases. Organisms tested included clostridia, anaerobic Gram-negative rods and the anaerobic cocci.

MATERIALS AND METHODS

All anaerobes in the study were first identified using routine laboratory methods (carbohydrate fermentation and GLC) (7).

Table 1. Enzyme substrates tested.

TEST NAME
1 Esterase C4
2 Naphthol-ASBi-phosphatase
3 β-glucuronidase
4 α-mannosidase
5 β-mannosidase
6 β-glucosidase
7 β-D-fucosidase
8 Trypsin
9 Leucine arylamidase
10 Valine arylamidase
11 Serine arylamidase
12 Lysine arylamidase
13 Hydroxyproline arylamidase
14 Aspartic arylamidase
15 Pyrrolidonic arylamidase
16 Phenylalanine arylamidase
17 Glutamylglutamic arylamidase
18 Lysylalanine arylamidase
19 Phenylalanine-arginine arylamidase
20 Proline-arginine arylamidase
21 Alkaline phosphatase
22 Acid phosphatase
23 Lipase CIO
24 α-Galactosidase
25 β-Galactosidase
26 α-Glucosidase
27 α-Fucosidase
28 L. Arabinosidase
29 Phospho-β-Galactosidase
30 N-Acetyl-β-glucosaminidase
31 Arginine arylamidase
32 Proline arylamidase
33 Ornithine arylamidase
34 Glutamine arylamidase
35 Histidine arylamidase
36 γ-glutamyl transpeptidase
37 Leucyl-glycine arylamidase
38 Histidyl-phenylalanine arylamidase
39 Glutamyl histidine arylamidase
40 Alanine-phenylalanine-proline arylamidase

For the enzyme tests the organisms were grown on
Columbia agar containing 5% horse blood for 48 hours
anaerobically. Suspensions of the organisms were made in
phosphate buffer (pH 7.2) equivalent to a McFarland
standard 5 or 6. 100 microlitres of this suspension was
added to 100 microlitres of substrate in appropriate wells
of a microtitre tray. The tray was covered and incubated
aerobically for 4 hours. All substrates were used at 0.2%
(w/v) concentration in phosphate buffer (pH 7.2). Table 1
lists the substrates used.

After 4 hr incubation at 37°C., activity of the carbohydrate glycosidases was observed by a change of the
solution in the well from colourless to bright yellow
indicating breakdown of the carbohydrate moeity and the
release of the ortho-nitrophenyl ion or p-nitrophenyl ion.

Formation of amino acid arylamidases were detected by
the addition of Zym A and Zym B reagent to the appropriate
wells. A positive result is detected by the formation of
a deep orange colour. Pale colour changes were disregarded.

```
Enzyme Reagent A
     Tris (hydroxymethyl) aminomethane    250 gm
     37% Hydrochloric acid                110 ml
     Lauryl sulphate                      100 gm
     Distilled water          to make   1,000 ml
                                        pH-7.6 - 7.8

Enzyme Reagent B
     Fast blue BB (Sigma F0250)           3.5 gm
     Z-methoxyethanol to make           1,000 ml
```

Indole production was detected by the addition of spot
indole reagent to the appropriate well. (Ehrlichs reagent
after xylene extraction is a suitable alternative).

```
Spot indole reagent
     P-dimethylaminocinnamaldehyde        1.0 gm
     10% (v/v) Conc Hydrochloric acid     100 ml
```

RESULTS

Nagler positive clostridia. *Clostridium perfringens* is an active carbohydrate fermenter and produces a wide range of glycosidases. The production of alpha and beta galactosidase differentiates this species from other

Table 2. Nagler positive Clostridia.

	C. bifermentans / sordellii	C. perfringens
Phosphatase	–	+
β – galactosidase	–	+
α – glucosidase	w	+
β – glucosidase	–	–
α – galactosidase	–	+
α – fucosidase	–	–
n-acetyl glucosaminidase	v	+
L-arabinosidase	–	–
β – glucuronidase	–	50
α – mannosidase	–	50
β – mannosidase	–	–
β – fucosidase	–	–
Indole	+	–
Leucine	–	–
Proline	+	–
Pyrroloidine	v	+

commonly encountered clostridia (*C. bifermentans* – *sordellii*) giving positive nagler reactions. Further promising tests for differentiation include the detection of a proline arylamidase. The appearance of two groups of *C. perfringens* is revealed by β –glucuronidase and α– manno-sidase activity.

Nagler negative clostridia. Good differentiation of the nagler negative clostridia encountered in our laboratory could be achieved using the glycoside substrates. Those species not producing these enzymes could be separated by examination of their arylamidase patterns. All strains of *C. difficile* failed to produce any glycosidases, but

consistently produced both a proline and a leucine arylamidase. *C. tetanii* gave negative profiles consistently.

Table 3. Nagler negative Clostridia.

	1	2	3	4	5	6
Phosphatase	–	–	–	–	–	–
β- galactosidase	–	–	–	–	–	–
α- glucosidase	–	+	–	+	w	–
β- glucosidase	–	+	–	–	w	–
α- galactosidase	–	+	–	–	–	–
α- fucosidase	+	–	–	–	–	–
n-acetyl glucosaminidase	+	–	–	+	–	–
L-arabinosidase	–	+	–	–	–	–
β- glucuronidase	–	–	–	–	–	–
α- mannosidase	–	–	–	–	–	–
β- mannosidase	–	–	–	–	–	–
β- fucosidase	–	–	–	+	–	–
Indole	+	–	–	–	–	+
Leucine	–	+	+	–	+	–
Proline	–	–	+	–	+	–
Pyrroloidine	+	–	–	–	50	–

1. *C. cadaveris*, 2. *C. chauveoi*, 3. *C. difficile*, 4. *C. septicum*,
5. *C. sporogenes*, 6. *C. tetani*

The Bacteroidaceae. Of the bacteroides and fusobacteria
the members of the "fragilis group" and *B. oralis* show the
most active glycosidase patterns. Differentiation of some
of the species within the "fragilis group" can be achieved.

> *B. distasonis* fails to elicit α-fucosidase
> *B. fragilis* fails to elicit L.-arabinosidase
> *B. vulgatus* fails to elicit β-glucosidase

Differentiation of the indole positive species has
proved more difficult. *B. uniformis* (not shown in the
table) can be differentiated from *B. thetaiotaomicron* and
B. ovatus by its failure to attack arginine and lysine.
It seems that a number of tests may be required to
separate *B. thetaiotaomicron* and *B. ovatus*. Arginine,
serine and histidine look promising in this respect.

Differentiation of *B. bivius* and *B. disiens* can be

Table 4.   The *Bacteroidacaea*.

	1	2	3	4	5	6	7
Phosphatase	+	+	+	+	+	+	+
β – galactosidase	+	+	+	+	+	+	+
α – glucosidase	+	+	+	+	+	+	+
β – glucosidase	+	+	+	+	–	–	–
α – galactosidase	+	+	+	+	+	–	–
α – fucosidase	–	+	+	+	+	+	–
n-acetyl-glucosaminidase	+	+	+	+	+	+	–
L-arabinosidase	+	–	+	+	+	–	–
Indole	–	–	+	+	–	–	–
Arginine AMP	+	+	–	–	+	(v)	+
Seryl AMP	+	+	–	v	v	–	v

1. *B.distasonis*, 2. *B.fragilis*, 3. *B.ovatus*, 4. *B.thetaiotaomicron*,
5. *B. vulgatus*, 6. *B. bivius*, 7. *B. disiens*

accomplished:-

(1) From each other by detection of α-fucosidase and N-acetylglucosaminidase.   *B. bivius* produces both enzymes but *B. disiens* fails to elicit either.

(2) From the fragilis group in their failure to produce

Table 5.   The *Bacteroidacaea*.

	1	2	3	4	5	6	7	8
Phosphatase	v	+	+	+	+	v	–	–
β – galactosidase	–	–	+	+	+	–	–	–
α – glucosidase	–	+	+	+	v	–	–	–
β – glucosidase	–	–	–	+	v	–	–	–
α – galactosidase	–	–	v	+	+	–	–	–
α – fucosidase	v	+	+	v	–	–	–	–
n-acetylglucosaminidase	–	–	+	+	–	–	–	–
L-arabinosidase	–	–	–	–	–	–	–	–
Indole	+	+	–	–	–	+	+	+
Arginine AMP	+	+	+	v	+	+	+	+
Seryl AMP	v	v	–	–	+	–	–	+
Pyrrolidonayl AMP						v	–	

1. *B. asaccharolyticus*, 2. *B. intermedius*, 3. *B. melaninogenicus*,
4. *B. oralis*, 5. *F. mortiferum*, 6. *F. necrophorum*, 7. *F. nucleatum*,
8. *F. varium*.

α-galactosidase.

Furthermore, *B. bivius* is almost always arginine arylamidase negative, whereas *B. melaninogenicus* strains that fail to elicit α-galactosidase are almost always arginine positive. Separation of the melaninogenicus group is possible using the combination of β-galactosidase, α-glucosidase and n-acetylglucosaminidase.

B.oralis has similar glucosidase patterns to *B.fragilis*. Seryl arylamidase, however, helps to differentiate these two organisms (*B. oralis* negative, *B. fragilis* positive). Further tests of help may include pyrrolidonyl, glutamyl-histidyl, glyceryl and phenylalanyl arylamidases.

Differentiation of the fusobacteria is more difficult. *F.mortiferum*, known to be a biochemically active member of the group, presents no difficulty. Differentiation of the other three commonly encountered fusobacteria is still problematical. *F.varium* produces both a serine and glycine arylamidase which may help in its recognition. Separation of *F.necrophorum* and *F.nucleatum* is much more difficult. Promising tests include P-nitrophenyl phosphatase, pyrrolidonyl arylamidase, acid and alkaline phosphatase and capric (decanoic) lipase.

A test for the combined production of alpha and beta glucosidase may prove promising in the differentiation of fusobacteria from bacteroides.

The anaerobic cocci. There still seems to be no one good test for the differentiation of the two main genera *Peptococcus* and *Peptostreptococcus*. Proline arylamidase may be the candidate we are looking for, as tests using this substrate look promising. So far, no strains of *Pc. asaccharolyticus*, *Pc. saccharolyticus Pc. magnus*, and *Pc. prevotii* and have produced this enzyme. All strains of *Pst. anaerobius* that we have examined so far have produced this enzyme as have the few strains of *Pst. micros*.

The finding of an anaerobic coccus producing only α-glucosidase and proline arylamidase is indicative of *Pst. anaerobius*. A wide glycosidase pattern could indicate *Pst. productus*.

Table 7. Anaerobic cocci.

	1	2	3	4	5	6
Phosphatase	−	+	−	−	−	−
β − galactosidase	−	−	+	−	−	−
α − glucosidase	+	−	+	−	−	−
β − glucosidase	−	−	−	−	−	−
α − galactosidase	−	−	+	−	−	−
α − fucosidase	−	−	−	−	−	−
n-acetyl glucosaminidase	−	−	−	−	−	−
L-arabinosidase	−	−	+	−	−	−
β − glucuronidase	−	−		−	−	−
α − mannosidase	−	−		−	−	−
β − mannosidase	−	−		−	−	−
β − fucosidase	−	−		−	−	−
Indole	−	−		+	−	−
Phenylanalyl AMP	−	+	−	+	+	−

1. *Pst. anaerobius*, 2. *Pst. micros*, 3. *Pst. productus*
4. *Pc. asaccharolyticus*, 5. *Pc. magnus*, 6. *Pc. prevotii*

Another problem in this group of anaerobes is the differentiation of the peptococci. Phenylalanine aryl-amidase seems to differentiate *Pc.magnus* from *Pc.prevotii*. Similarly, pyrrolidine arylamidase may also be helpful.

DISCUSSION

The standard methods for the identification of clinically important anaerobic bacteria are time consuming and it is normally some days after the beginning of treat-ment of the patient that an identification of the organism is available to the clinician. If identification schemes for anaerobes are to be more valuable then there is a clear need for more rapid techniques to be developed. Work along this path has led to the use of the API ZYM strip which has proved useful (6, 8). However, we feel that there is a need for a more specific set (or sets) of enzyme tests. Work using carbohydrate glycosidases has proved useful for differentiating different groups of bacteria (4, 5). According to Tharagonnet et al (6) some encouraging results were obtained within the *Bacteroidaceae* and subspeciation of the *B. melaninogenicus* group could be achieved. Results in this study further support their findings. We have also shown that differentiation of *B.bivius* from non-pigmented *B.melaninogenicus* is also possible using the system reported here. We also show here that rapid recognition of certain members within the "*B.fragilis*" group, *B. bivius*, *B. disiens*, *B. oralis*, and some of the fusobacteria can be performed with good reproducibility and accuracy.

A further encouraging finding is the possibility of differentiating the two genera *Bacteroides* and *Fusobacterium*. Work will continue on this interesting aspect of the study.

Early recognition of clinically important clostridia was achieved. Results with *C. difficile* were particularly specific and this may be an advantage for those laboratories who do not have access to a gas liquid chromatograph. We do not yet know the significance of the two glycosidase patterns given by strains of *C. perfringens*.

Differentiation of commonly encountered anaerobic cocci was obtained and shows the advantage of such a system where many strains are asaccharolytic in conventional identification schemes. The separation of peptococci and peptostreptococci is a distinct possibility with the system. Further strains, however, need to be tested.

We conclude that rapid enzyme testing provides an alternative technique for the identification of clinically important anaerobic bacteria. Advantages of such a system include speed of identification and the differentiation of hitherto similar asaccharolytic species.

References

1   Holdeman, L.V., and Moore, W.E.C. (1977). Anaerobic Laboratory Manual, Virginia Polytechnic Institute & State University, Blacksburg, Virginia.(4th Edition)

2   Sutter, V., Citron, D., and Finegold, S.M. 1980. Wadsworth Anaerobe Bacteriology Manual, C.V. Mosby Co. (3rd edition).

3   Westley, J.W., Anderson, P.J., Close, V.A., Halpern, B., and Lederberg, E.M. 1967. Aminopeptidase profiles of various bacteria. Appl. Microbiol. 15: 822-825.

4   Kilian, M. and Bulow, P. 1976. Rapid detection and identification of Enterobacteriaceae. Acta. Path. Microbiol. Scand. 54: 245-251.

5   Kilian, M. 1978. Rapid identification of Actinomycetaceae and related bacteria. J. Clin. Microbiol. 8: 127-133.

6   Tharagonnet, D., Sisson, P.R., Roxby, C.M., Ingham, H.R. and Selkon, J.B. 1977. The API ZYM system in the identification of Gram-negative anaerobes. J. Clin. Pathol. 30: 505-509.

7   Wren, M.W.D. 1980. Prolonged primary incubation in the isolation of anaerobic bacteria from clinical specimens. J. Med. Microbiol. 13: 257-263.

8   Marler, L., Allen, S., & Siders. J. 1984. Rapid enzymatic characterization of clinically encountered anaerobic bacteria with the API ZYM system. Euro. J. Clin. Microbiol. 3: 294-300.

CHAPTER 3

SENSITIVITY TESTING AND MIC DETERMINATION
OF OBLIGATE ANAEROBES

D.Felmingham

Department of Clinical Microbiology, University College
Hospital, Gower Street, London, WC1, UK.

Contents

Abstract

Many clinical laboratories do not investigate the antimicrobial susceptibility of clinical isolates of obligately anaerobic bacteria routinely, relying instead on the pan-antimicrobial spectrum of metronidazole or on published susceptibility profiles often determined with organisms isolated from patients at other, widely distant, hospitals. This approach can be seriously questioned in the light of increasing evidence of regional variation in antimicrobial susceptibility patterns which may reflect local prescribing habits.

The major reason for the reluctance of laboratories to investigate obligately anaerobic bacteria with the same, often irrelevant, enthusiasm shown for other organisms appears to be the generally held view that susceptibility testing and Minimum Inhibitory Concentration (MIC) determination are both more difficult to perform and the results less valid than those obtained, using similar techniques, with facultatively anaerobic and aerobic isolates. The basic problem, particularly with disc diffusion sensitivity testing, is the relatively slow growth rate of many obligately anaerobic bacteria on media commonly employed for sensitivity testing and MIC determination.

SECTION 2. ANAEROBES AND GASTROINTESTINAL DISEASE

Chairman of Session : Dr. B.S. Drasar

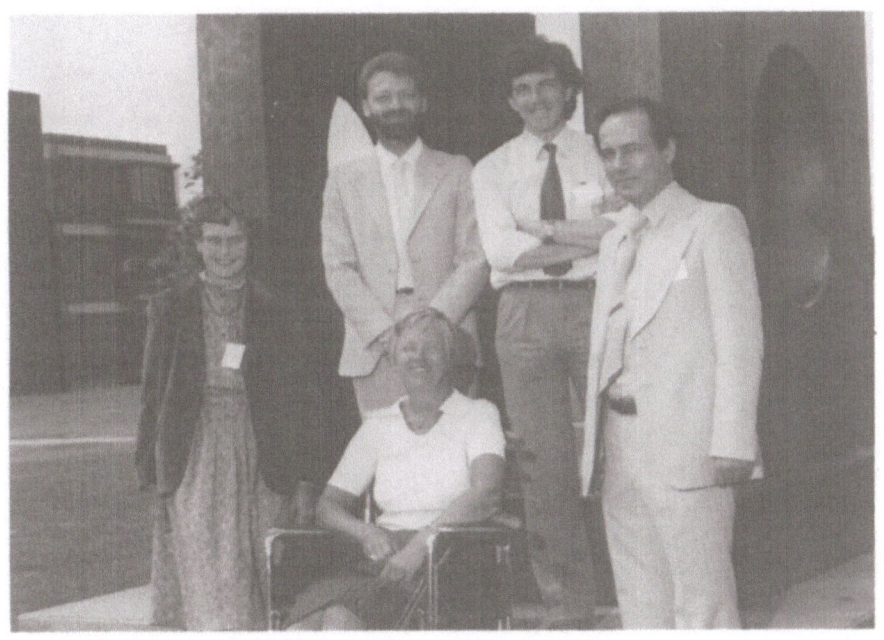

From left to right :-

Standing : Jean M. Dolby, S.P. Borriello, M.J. Hudson and B.S. Drasar

Seated : Kari Hovind-Hougen.

CHAPTER 4

CLOSTRIDIUM PERFRINGENS ENTEROTOXIN-ASSOCIATED DIARRHOEA

S.P. Borriello, H.E. Larson, Fiona E. Barclay and A.R. Welch

Division of Communicable Diseases, Clinical Research Centre, Watford Road, Harrow, Middlesex, HA1 3UJ, England.

Contents

Abstract

Introduction

Pathogenesis

Associated features

Epidemiology

Treatment and management

Concluding remarks

References

ABSTRACT

Enterotoxigenic strains of *C. perfringens* are now
implicated in cases of diarrhoea other than food poisoning.
There is good evidence that cross-infection may occur and
that cross-infection control measures are helpful in
limiting spread of the disease. The organism can be
readily isolated from the immediate environment of
affected patients as well as from their hands. In general
the diarrhoea is self limiting, but metronidazole or
vancomycin may be used to treat troublesome cases. Faecal
blood and mucous and abdominal pain feature in about half
of the cases.

INTRODUCTION

Diarrhoea is still one of the major causes of mortality
and morbidity in the world, causing over 10 million deaths
per year. Although new aetiological agents such as
Clostridium difficile *and* Aeromonas *sp. have recently been*
identified, there are still many cases of diarrhoea where
an established causal agent can not be implicated. There
are, of course, a number of changes in the gut flora,
especially following antimicrobial therapy, that would
account for this problem in some cases, even in the
absence of a specific pathogen (2). However, as well as
cases totally unrelated to the gut flora, other pathogenic
micro-organisms must account for some cases. We have
recently shown that enterotoxigenic strains of *Clostridium
perfringens* are one such candidate (5).

Although the role of *C. perfringens* in food poisoning

has long been known, its role in diarrhoea unrelated to food poisoning was not established until our recent work implicating *C. perfringens* in antibiotic-associated diarrhoea (5). Since this initial description of eleven patients, a further 32 cases have been detected. The clinical and microbiological findings in these patients will be presented.

PATHOGENESIS

A cytotoxin, other than that of *C. difficile*, was found in faecal specimens during a recent investigation of patients with antibiotic-associated diarrhoea. This faecal cytotoxin was identified as *C. perfringens* enterotoxin by neutraliz-ation tests with specific antitoxin in tissue culture and by an enzyme-linked immunoassay (5). In addition very high numbers of enterotoxigenic *C. perfringens* were detected in the stools of all patients when toxin was present but in only about half of control patients, who also carried far fewer organisms (5).

Since this description of eleven patients a further thirty-two have been detected. In keeping with our earlier findings in many of them (60%) the diarrhoea was

Table 1. Antibiotics associated with *C. perfringens* diarrhoea

	Alone	In combination	Total
Amoxacillin	3	3	6
Flocloxacillin	1	4	5
Ampicillin	2	1	3
Penicillin	1	2	3
Cefuroxime	2	1	3
Co-trimoxazole	2	1	3
Trimethoprim	2	0	2
Cephalexin	0	2	2
Nystatin, piperacillin, augmentin	1	0	3
Tobramycin, gentamicin, metronidazole	0	1	3
Unknown			5
None			15

antibiotic-associated (Table 1).

Not all cases however, are associated with antibiotics, and it is also evident that *C. perfringens* may be an important cause of sporadic diarrhoea. In those antibiotic-associated cases the apparent association with the penicillins noted in the earlier study (5) is still apparent in this extended series of patients. This is of particular interest in view of the reports of acute colitis related to penicillin and its derivatives (1,9,10) where cases were characterised by a self limiting diarrhoea in which there was abdominal pain, faecal blood but normal rectal mucosa. However, abnormalities were noted in the proximal large bowel. Two of these reports pre-date our knowledge of the involvement of *C. difficile* in disease (1,10) and the other report failed to look for cytotoxins or *C. difficile*. Although *C. difficile* could have played a role in the disease, the findings of pain, blood and normal rectum, as well as the absence of pseudomembranes in the gut, are much more consistent with a possible involvement of enterotoxigenic *C.perfringens*, which shares many of these features (see below). The frequency of blood and mucous in the stools of patients with *C. perfringens* diarrhoea (Table 2) coupled to a relatively

Table 2. Features of 43 cases of *C. perfringens* diarrhoea

Observation	No. of patients where information available	Mean (range)
$\log_2$ toxin titre/g. faeces	42	9.4 (4–17)
$\log_{10}$ No. *C. perfringens*/g. faeces	43	8.4 (7. 0–10. 3)
Bowel motions/day	33	5.7 (1–20)
Duration of diarrhoea (days)	34	10.5 (2–50) days
Days since antibiotic withdrawn	20	1 1. 7 (0–48) days
White cells/ml of blood	24	9.9 (3. 1–34.6) x10^3
Age (years)	43	76.4 (25–99)

normal rectal mucosa may be indicative of more proximal large bowel involvement.

It is likely that small bowel colonization with *C. perfringens* is necessary for disease, as it is believed that the site of action of the enterotoxin for the induction of net secretion is in the small bowel, the toxin having no measurable effect in the colon of the rabbit (8). This may help to explain treatment success with metronidazole (see below) despite failure to significantly reduce faecal levels of the causative enterotoxigenic serotype. In this case it is probable that treatment removed *C. perfringens* from the small bowel.

ASSOCIATED FEATURES

The features associated with *C. perfringens* diarrhoea are listed in Tables 2 and 3. As can be seen, very high levels of enterotoxin, up to a titre of 1:128,000, and high numbers of *C. perfringens*, up to 10^{10} per gram, may be present. There is, however, no direct correlation between enterotoxin titre and numbers of *C. perfringens*.

Table 3. Features of 43 cases of *C. perfringens* diarrhoea

Observation	No. of patients where information available	No. positive (%)
Antibiotic associated	38	23 (60%)
Vomiting	29	6 (21%)
Abdominal pain	35	18 (51%)
Blood or mucous in faeces	36	18 (50%)
Other pathogens identified	34	4 (12%)

The diarrhoea tends to be fluid and foul smelling, lasting on average for eleven days, although affecting some people for prolonged periods. Most patients pass between four and ten motions a day but in some cases the diarrhoea is both profuse and continuous. Both blood and mucous are frequently present in the stools and over half of the patients have abdominal pain, which can be severe. There is however, no direct correlation between blood and mucous and abdominal pain. In general there is no elevation of numbers of white blood cells. Up to one fifth of patients experience vomiting, all but one of these patients also had abdominal pain. In general the patients affected with *C. perfringens* diarrhoea are old. This may be because they are more susceptible to colonization with this organism. In support of this argument are the findings of Yamagishi and colleagues (12) demonstrating persistent carriage of high numbers of *C. perfringens* in healthy institution- alised geriatrics.

The only consistent histological finding from analysis of rectal biopsies obtained at sigmoidoscopy is that of oedema.

In only four cases has another possible pathogen been isolated from the faeces, and in all four cases it was *C. difficile*. However, in three of these cases the *C. difficile* isolates were non-toxigenic. In one case, however, both toxigenic *C. difficile* and *C. perfringens* were isolated and both *C. difficile* cytotoxin and *C. perfringens* enterotoxin were detected in the stool (6).

EPIDEMIOLOGY

There is now good evidence of case-clustering associated with a common serotype of enterotoxigenic *C. perfringens* (4, 11). During one of these case clusters affecting five geriatric patients over a nine week period, with four of the cases occurring over two weeks, an exten- sive epidemiological survey was performed. It was shown that the outbreak serotype of *C. perfringens* was rarely present in the faeces of asymptomatic patients on the same ward as affected patients. It could be isolated from the hands of patients with the disease and occasionally from the hands of staff dealing with these patients (3, 4). It also could be readily isolated from the inanimate surfaces in the immediate environment of patients with *C. perfringens* diarrhoea but not from similar areas for a patient with *C. difficile* mediated diarrhoea. The results of environmental sampling in single rooms and on general wards are presented in Table 4. The rate of isolation halved once the diarrhoea had resolved, and the causative serotype was rarely isolated from areas where there was no known history of the disease. It is evident that extensive environmental contamination may take place and that viable spores may survive for some time in the environment, which contributes to the risk of cross infection. It is likely that enterotoxigenic strains of *C. perfringens* may cause cross-infection in much the same way as *C. difficile*.

Table 4. Prevalence in the environment of the *C. perfringens* causing diarrhoea.

	Wards	Sluice
Active disease	69%	39%
Previous active disease	29%	12.5%
No disease	11%	0%

TREATMENT AND MANAGEMENT

There is little information available on treatment (7). Most of the patients described by Borriello and colleagues (5) had self limiting diarrhoea, even though in some cases the diarrhoea was protracted. One of the patients was treated with vancomycin but relapsed after treatment (5), (the same serotype of *C. perfringens* causing the relapse). One patient improved without further complication after administration of codeine (5). In general treatment is supportive, however, due to the severity of the diarrhoea, it has proven necessary to treat four patients. Three responded within 36 hours to treatment with metronidazole (400 mg three times daily, orally for 7 days) and one patient failed to respond (11). In the one patient studied in detail, a very good relationship was shown between metronidazole therapy and the concomitant resolution of symptoms, decrease in the numbers of *C. perfringens* and disappearance of enterotoxin from the faeces (7).

It is evident from the epidemiological studies (see above) that spread of infection is probably by the faecal oral route. It would seem sensible to implement some sort of cross-infection control measures. It was possible to control a recent outbreak of this diarrhoea by isolating affected patients to one part of a ward and using cohort nursing and separate toilet and washing facilities (11). This procedure obviated the requirement for formal isolation facilities which are expensive and stressful to elderly patients.

CONCLUDING REMARKS

The evidence to date implies that enterotoxigenic strains of *C. perfringens* behave as a true infectious agent, in much the same way as *C. difficile*, and that implementation of cross-infection control measures are important in limiting spread of the disease. In the majority of cases the diarrhoea is self limiting and specific therapy is not required. For problematic cases metronidazole or vancomycin may be useful.

References

1   Barrison, I.G. and Kane, S.P.   1978.   Penicillin-
     associated colitis.   Lancet 2:   843.

2   Borriello, S.P. 1984. Bacteria and gastrointestinal
     secretion and motility.
     Scand. J. Gastroenterol.   19: 115-121.

3   Borriello, S.P.   1985.   Newly described clostridial
     diseases of the gastrointestinal tract: *Clostridium
     perfringens* enterotoxin-associated diarrhoea and
     neutropenic enterocolitis due to Clostridium
     septicum.   In: S.P. Borriello (ed).   Clostridial
     Diseases of the Gastrointestinal Tract.   CRC Press
     Inc. Florida.   p.   223.

4   Borriello, S.P., Barclay, F.E., Welch, A.R.,
     Stringer, M.F., Watson, G.N., Williams, R.K.T., Seal,
     D.V. and Sullens, K.   1985.   Epidemiology of
     diarrhoea caused by enterotoxigenic *Clostridium
     perfringens*.   J.   Med. Microbiol.   20: 363-372

5   Borriello, S.P., Larson, H.E., Welch, A.R., Barclay,
     F., Stringer, M.F. and Bartholomew, B.A.   1984.
     Enterotoxigenic *Clostridium perfringens*: A possible
     cause of antibiotic-associated diarrhoea.
     Lancet 1:   305-307.

6   Borriello, S.P., Welch, A.R., Larson, H.E. and
     Barclay, F.E. 1984.   Diarrhoea and simultaneous
     excretion of *Clostridium difficile* cytotoxin and
     C.perfringens enterotoxin.   Lancet.   2: 1218.

7   Borriello, S.P. and Williams R.K.T.   1985.   Treatment
     of *Clostridium perfringens* enterotoxin-associated
     diarrhoea with metronidazole.   J.infect. 10:   65-67.

8   McDonel, J.L. and Demers, G.W.   1982.   *In vivo*
     effects of enterotoxin from *Clostridium perfringens*
     Type A in the rabbit colon: Binding vs. biological
     activity.   J. Infect. Dis.   145:   490-494

9   Sakurai. Y., Tsuchiya, H., Ikegami, F., Funatomi, T.,
     Takasu, S. and Uchikoshi, T. 1979. Acute right-sided
     hemorrhagic colitis associated with oral
     administration of ampicillin.
     Dig.   Dis. Sci.   24: 910-915.

10   Toffler, R.B., Pingoud, E.G. and Burrell, M.I.
     1978.   Acute colitis related to penicillin and
     penicillin derivatives.   Lancet 2:   707-709.

11   Williams, R., Piper, M., Boriello, S.P., Barclay, F.,
     Welch, A., Seal, D. and Sullens, K. 1985.   Diarrhoea
     due to entero-toxigenic *Clostridium perfringens*:
     Clinical features and management of a cluster of 10
     cases.   Age and ageing 14:   296-302.

12   Yamagishi, T., Serikawa, T., Morita, R., Nakamura, S.
     and Nishida, S.   1976.   Persistent high numbers of
     Clostridium perfringens in the intestines of Japanese
     aged adults. Jap. J.   Microbiol. 20: 397-403.

CHAPTER 5

GASTROINTESTINAL CAMPYLOBACTER-LIKE ORGANISMS

Jean M. Dolby

Division of Communicable Diseases, Clinical Research Centre,
Harrow, Middlesex, HA1 3UJ, U.K.

Contents

Abstract

Introduction

C. *Fetus* and C. *jejunii* and other thermophilic
    diarrhoea-producing campylobacters.

Gastric and duodenal ulcers, gastritis
    and C. *'pylorodis'*

Other CLO's

Conclusions

References

ABSTRACT

Campylobacter jejuni, the aetiological agent of 5-10% of episodes of diarrhoea in North America and Europe is described and its relatives *C. coli* and *C. laridis* are mentioned; and are compared with *C.fetus*. The predilection of campylobacters for immuno-compromised hosts is discussed.

Organisns similar to these and called campylobacter-like (CLO) have been described recently. *C. 'pyloridis'* or G.CLO-1, the best known, is isolated from the antrum of the stomach in close association with gastritis and gastric and duodenal ulcers. Its properties are compared with those of *C. jejuni*. Another stomach isolate in association with gastritis is G.CLO-2. From hypogamma-globulinaemic patients an organism very similar to *C. 'pyloridis'* has been found. This differs in being resistant to erythromycin. It also produces less acidic mucosubstance *in vitro* than does *C. 'pyloridis'*, whereas G.CLO-2 produces a similar amount and *C. jejuni* none. *C. 'cinaedi'* and *C. 'fennelliae'* have been isolated from rectal biopsies of male patients with proctitis and diarrhoea and *C. 'cinaedi'* from the blood of immune-compromised male homosexuals. *C. 'hyointestinalis'* isolated from prolifer-ative enteritis in pigs is the only facul-tative anaerobe, all the other organisms described as being microaerophilic. Plating of filtered specimens onto antibiotic-free media have yielded other CLOs associated with diarrhoea.

INTRODUCTION

I propose to give a review of this rapidly expanding

group of organisms, including our own work where relevant, but relying much on that of others, to provide some footholds for the new literature. The proceedings of the Third International Workshop on Campylobacter Infections (23) will provide information on current work and a bibliography for those further interested. I shall begin by describing briefly the known thermophilic (ie. ability to grow at 42°C.) diarrhoea-producing campylobacters and *C. fetus* for comparison and then go onto the newer campylobacter-like organisms (CLOs).

C. FETUS AND *C. JEJUNI* AND OTHER THERMOPHILIC DIARRHOEA-PRODUCING CAMPYLOBACTERS

C. jejuni was described in stools of diarrhoea patients in 1957 by Elizabeth King who referred to it as a vibrio-related organism, comparing it with *Vibrio fetus* which causes infertility in cattle. Isolation and growth had to wait until the application of procedures ie. filtration of stools, microaerophilic conditions and selective media, by a Belgian team. The results were published in 1972. A young member of that team, now Professor Butzler, extended this work, and he in Belgium and Dr. Skirrow in this country, showed that 5-10% of all diarrhoeas were due to this organism, which was put into a new genus *Campylobacter* and called *C. jejuni* (3). Also transferred into this genus were *Vibrio fetus* (which became *C. fetus*), *C. coli*, and the naladixic acid resistant, thermophilic campylobacter (NARTC) *C. laridis* (2). Infections are usually food-borne or acquired from pets and the causative organisms are isolated from poultry, milk and water. Successful epidemiology has depended on the use of selective blood agar containing appropriate antibiotics, eg. vancomycin, trimethoprin and polymyxin B (26).

C. jejuni accounts for most of the campylobacter diarrhoea: *C. coli*, *C. fetus* (24) and *C. laridis* (29) are found infrequently. *C. fetus* is the campylobacter most often isolated from the blood stream. Although *C. jejuni* becomes transiently blood-borne 24-48 hours following intestinal infection, its isolation from the blood is rare. It has long been known that *C. fetus* causes generalised systemic infection, frequently fatal, in immuno-compromised hosts.

C. jejuni diarrhoea is usually a 5-10 day, self-limiting but often quite severe disease in normal hosts, sometimes with blood and mucus in the stools (26). In hypogammaglobulinaemic patients diarrhoea may be severe and chronic it being possible to make repeated isolations of the same serotype of *C. jejuni* (11). Six patients at Northwick Park hospital have had diarrhoea, however without any campylobacters or other intestinal pathogens being isolated. Campylobacter could be demonstrated in their faeces, however, using a recently developed immunofluorescent technique (21). The test is dependent on a heat-stable antigen which cross-reacts with *C. coli*, *C. laridis* and some of the CLOs. We believe, therefore, that those patients may carry CLOs. This finding suggested that more campylobacters could be isolated under the right conditions.

Pathogenic gastro-intestinal campylobacters are catalase-positive, oxidase-positive, small, curved, flagellated Gram-negative rods growing microaerophilically (27). A catalase-negative campylobacter *C. sputorum* sub-species *mucosalis* has been demonstrated intra-cellularly in a proliferative enteritis of pigs but whether it is the casual agent has yet to be proven. Several species grow

Table 1. Some properties of known campylobacters compared with G.CLO-1

Organism	Growth at °C 43	Growth at °C 37	Growth at °C 25	NA* (30 mcg)	H₂S	Hydrol. hipp.	Urease
C. fetus	−	+	+	R	−	−	−
Atypical C. fetus	+	+	+	R	−	−	−
C. jejuni I	+	+	−	S	−	+	−
C. jejuni II	+	+	−	S	+	+	−
C. coli	+	+	−	S	−	−	−
C. laridis	+	+	−	R	+	−	−
C. 'pyloridis' (G. CLO-1)	−	+	−	R	+	−	

* Naladixic acid resistance (R) and sensitivity (S)

at 42°C. They do not ferment carbohydrates and are distinguished by tests shown in Tables 1 and 2. Some of these tests need experience in interpretation and reliance is placed on DNA homology and hybridisation tests for confirming similarities and differences, particularly of newer CLOs (1, 17).

Most work has been done on C. jejuni. Using an extensive enzyme testing system (4) biotypes of it and of C. coli have now been described (25). There are over 40 serotypes determined by the lipopolysaccharide antigen (20) and more than 60 based on heat-labile antigens (12). The organism has two flagella, one at each end: the flagellar protein is a major outer membrane protein (OMP) component running at 62K by SDS-PAGE (16). The main antibody response in convalescent humans following infection is to this antigen (31) although it is probably not the protective antibody (4).

Table 1 shows some of the biochemical properties of

C. jejuni compared with *C. fetus*, *C. laridis* and *C. coli*. Recently an atypical *C. fetus* has been discovered growing at 42°C. (5). It has been common practice to isolate all campylobacters on selective media. A return to the practice of filtration through an 0.65 micrometre membrane onto fresh blood agar has yielded an antibiotic-sensitive strain of *C. jejuni* and a new CLO with only a weak catalase reaction which has been found (particularly) in young children with diarrhoea in Australia (28).

Table 2. Properties of Campylobacter-like organisms (CLOs)

Organism Code/sp. nov.			Growth 42°C	NA[1]	Hydrol. Hipp. HH[2]	Red. No3 NR[3]	Flagella
C.pyloridis G. CLO-1	))	Gastritis Stomach	−	R	−	−	4 − 5 unipolar
G. CLO-2		Gastritis Stomach	−	S	+	−/wk	1
CLO-1 *C.cinaedi*	))	Proctitis Rectum	−	S	−	+	1
CLO-2 *C.fennelliae*	))	Proctitis Rectum	−	S	−	−	1
CLO-3		Proctitis	+	S	−	−	1
H. CLO-1		Immunodefic. Blood	−	S	−	+	1
C.hyointestinalis		Prolif. ent. (Pigs)	+	R	−	+	1

[1] Naladixic acid resistance R (or sensitive S) to 30 mcg/ml antibiotic
[2] Hydrolysis of Hippurate
[3] Nitrate Reduction

GASTRIC and DUODENAL ULCERS, GASTRITIS and *C.'PYLORODIS'*

   C. 'pyloridis' is perhaps the most well-known of the new CLOs. Two years ago Warren and Marshall reported that the small spiral organisms observed for many years by histologists in stomach biopsies of patients with gastritis and peptic ulcer disease had at last been grown from stomach biopsies in the microbiology laboratory of the Royal Perth Hospital of Western Australia. The organism was identified as a campylobacter (G. CLO-1) and the species name pyloridis suggested (14). It is more fragile than *C. jejuni*. It requires fresh, moist medium and a longer incubation time of 4-6 days. It will grow on *C. jejuni*-selective medium but not at 42°C and is characterised by a strong urease (18). Growth from gastric tissue (for which it has a specificity) is associated with gastritis and peptic ulcer disease (22). Serum antibody from this organism as detected by complement fixation is elevated in patients with these conditions (6). An animal model is not yet available but an attempt to fulfil Koch's postulates in a human volunteer is reported (13).

Morphologically the organism is distinct from *C.jejuni* and other campylobacters in having up to five unipolar flagellae, which are sheathed and bulbous ended (9). The molecular weight of flagellar protein is lower than that for *C. jejuni*; there is no major OMP and total protein profiles of several strains are similar to each other but different from other campylobacters (15). There is no evidence of a multiplicity or serotypes although surface proteins may be distinctive. The methylated esters of cellular fatty acids of this organism are distinctive from those of *C. jejuni* (9).

OTHER CLOs

From the stomachs of six patients with gastritis amongst 300 studied in a German clinic, another strain called G.CLO-2 has been isolated (10). It has one flagellum, is more robust than *C. 'pyloridis'*, urease negative and is more like *C. jejuni* in many respects: it fails to grow at 42°C, but it hydrolyses hippurate. Its properties are shown in Table 2 compared with other CLOs.

Three strains, CLO 1-3 have been isolated from rectal biopsies of male patients with proctitis and diarrhoea and characterised (7). One of these, initially called H.CLO-1, was isolated from the blood of two homosexual male patients who were immunosuppressed (19). It has been shown to be the same as CLO-1. It and CLO-2 have now been provisionally named (30), as shown in Table 2.

The only non-human strain in Table 2 is *C. 'hyointestinalis'* which like *C. mucosalis* was isolated from lesions of prolif-erative enteritis in pigs (8): it has also been found in the stools of cattle and one hamster. This organism will grow well anaerobically as well as

Table 3. DNA composition of campylobacters

Organism	Mol% G + C*	Anaerobic Growth
C. jejuni	31	−
C. coli	31	−
C. fetus	34	±
Atypical *C. fetus*	34	±
C. 'pyloridis'	36-37	−
G. CLO-2	29	−
C. 'cinaedi'	37-38	−
C. 'fennelliae'	37	−
CLO-3	45	−
C. 'hyointestinalis'	36	+

* The base-pair ratios, guanine and cytosine are collected from sources describing individual organisms cited in the text.

microaerophilically and is the only CLO so far discovered
to do so.

DNA studies have justified the separation of these
organisms into species, as shown in Table 3. The atypical
C. fetus growing at 42°C. matches *C. fetus* G.CLO-2
more like *C. jejuni* than *C. 'pyloridis'* in many properties
is also more like it in this respect. CLO-3 has a very
high G+C ratio and may not be a campylobacter.

From gastric antral biopsy tissue and gastric juice of
two hypogammoglobulinaemic patients, we have now grown
another organism very like *C. 'pyloridis'*. Such patients
had typical atrophic gastritis (G. Slavin unpub.) but not
diarrhoea. Distinctions from *C. 'pyloridis'* are its
resistance to erythromycin, which is possibly because of

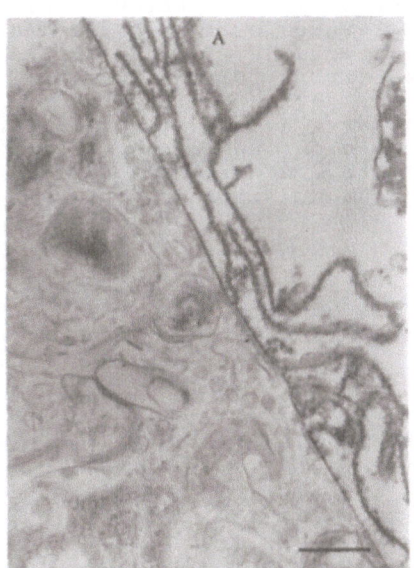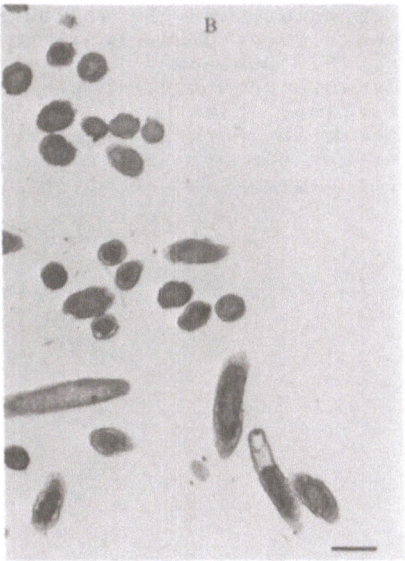

Figure 1. Ultrathin sections of bacterial colonies, on agar,
treatment with ruthenium red at primary and post-fixation
stages to show presence or absence of acidic mucosubstances at
colony surfaces which run diagonally from top-left to bottom-
right of print. Bars represent 500nm.
a) *C.'pyloridis'*; b) *C.jejuni*

frequent exposure, and the apparent production *in vitro* of much less or different specific acid mucosubstance stained by ruthenium red in electron micrographs, *C. 'pyloridis'* produces much of this substance *in vitro* (Figure 1a), *C. jejuni* by comparison produces none (Figure 1b).

CONCLUSION

The campylobacters can colonise the gastrointestinal tract. Whether the presence of the newer ones contribute to or cause disease, or whether they are opportunistic does perhaps require more than Dr. Marshall's one brave 'experiment' (13). The next few years will prove exciting particularly in the field of immunology and the role host defences play in infection and recovery.

ACKNOWLEDGEMENTS

The author thanks the organisers of the Anaerobe Discussion Group for the opportunity to present this information and the following colleagues with whom it has been a great pleasure to collaborate: Dr. A.B. Price, Mr. P. Dunscombe, Dr. A. Smith, Mr. J. Clark, Mrs. H.A. Davies, Dr. A.D.B. Webster, Dr. D.V. Seal, Miss J. Stirling, Miss M. L. Stephenson, Mrs. A.G. Hassan, all of Northwick Park Hospital or the Clinical Research Centre, Harrow and Dr. D.G. Newell, PHLS, Centre for Applied Microbiology and Research, Porton Down, Wiltshire.

References

1   Belland, R.J. and Trust, T.J. 1982.
Deoxyribonucleic acid sequence relatedness between
thermophilic members of the genus *Campylobacter*.
J. Gen. Microbiol. 128: 2515-2522.

2   Benjamin, J., Leaper, S., Owen, R.J. and Skirrow,
M.B. 1983. Description of *Campylobacter laridis*, a
new species comprising the nalidixic acid resistant,
thermophilic campylobacter (NARTC) group.
Curr. Microbiol. 8: 231-238.

3   Butzler, J.P. and Skirrow, M.B. 1979. *Campylobacter
enteritis*. Clin. Gastroenterol. 8: 737-765.

4   Dolby, J.M. and Newell, D,G. 1986. The protection
of infant mice from colonisation with *Campylobacter
jejuni* by vaccination of the dams.
Submitted to J. Hyg. Camb.

5   Edmonds, P., Patton, C.M., Barrett, T.J., Morris,
G.K., Steigerwalt, A.G. and Brenner, D.J. 1985.
Biochemical and genetic characteristics of atypical
Campylobacter fetus subsp. *fetus* strains isolated
from humans in the United States.
J. Clin. Microbiol. 21: 936-940.

6   Eldrige, J., Lessells, A.M. and Jones, D.M. 1984.
Antibody to spiral organisms on gastric mucosa.
Lancet 1, 1237.

7   Fennell, C.L., Totten, P.A., Quinn, T.C,, Patton,
D.L., Holmes, K.K. and Stamm, W.E. 1984.
Characterisation of Campylobacter-like organisms
isolated from homosexual men.
J. Infect. Dis. 149: 58-66.

8   Gebhart, C.J., Edmonds, P., Ward, G.E., Kurtz, H.J.
and Brenner, D.J. 1985. "*Campylobacter hyointestinalis*"
sp. nov.: a new species of Campylobacter found in
the intestines of pigs and other animals.
J. Clin. Microbiol. 21: 715-720.

9   Goodwin, C.S., McCullogh, R.K., Armstrong, J.A. and
Wee, S.H. 1985. Unusual cellular fatty acids and
distinctive ultrastructure in a new spiral bacterium
(*Campylobacter pyloridis*) from the human gastric
mucosa. J. Med. Microbiol. 19: 257-267.

10   Kasper, G. and Dickgiesser, N. 1985. Isolation from
gastric epithelium of campylobacter-like bacteria
that are distinct from "*Campylobacter pyloridis*".
Lancet 1: 111-112.

11   Lever, A., Dolby, J.M., Webster, A.D.B. and Price,
A.B. 1984. Chronic campylobacter colitis and
uveitis in patients with hypogammaglobulinaemia.
British Medical Journal 1: 531.

54

12   Lior, H., Woodward, D.L., Edgar, J.A., Leroche, L.J.
      and Gill, P. 1982. Serotyping of *Campylobacter
      jejuni* by slide agglutination based on heat-labile
      antigenic factors. J. Clin. Microbiol. 15: 761-768.

13   Marshall, B.J., Armstrong, J.A., McGechie, D.B. and
      Glancy, R.J. 1985. Attempt to fulfil Koch's
      postulates for pyloric campylobacter.
      Med. J. Australia 142: 436-439.

14   Marshall, B.J. and Warren, J.R. 1984. Unidentified
      curved bacilli in the stomach of patients with
      gastritis and peptic ulceration.
      Lancet 1: 1311-1314.

15   Newell, D.G. 1985. The outer membrane proteins and
      surface antigens of *C.pyloridis*. In: A.D. Pearson,
      M.B. Skirrow, H. Lior and B. Rowe (eds.)
      Campylobacter III,   Proceedings,   Third
      International Workshop on Campylobacter infections.
      (in press)

16   Newell, D.G., McBride, H. and Pearson, A.D.   1984.
      The identification of outer membrane proteins and
      flagella of *Campylobacter jejuni*.
      J. Gen. Microbiol. 130: 1201-1208.

17   Owen, R.J.   1983. Nucleic acids in the classifi-
      cation of campylobacters.
      Europ. J. Clin. Microbiol. 2: 367-377.

18   Owen, R.J., Martin, S.R. and Borman, P. 1985.
      Rapid urea hydrolysis by gastric campylobacters.
    Lancet 1: 111.

19   Pasternak, J., Bolivar, R., Hopfer, R.L., Fainstein,
      V., Mills, K., Rios, A., Bodey, G.P., Fennell, C.L.,
      Totten, P.A. and Stamm, W. E. 1984. Bacteraemia
      caused by Campylobacter-like organisms in two male
      homosexuals. Ann. Intern. Med. 101: 339-341.

20   Penner, J.L. and Hennessy, J.M.   1980.   Passive
      haemagglutination technique for serotyping
      Campylobacter fetus subsp. *jejuni* on the basis of
      soluble heat-stable   antigens.
      J. Clin. Microbiol. 12: 732-737.

21   Price, A.B., Dolby J.M., Dunscombe, P.R., and
      Stirling, J.   1984. Detection of campylobacter by
      immunofluorescence in stools and rectal biopsies of
      patients with diarrhoea.
      J. Clin. Pathol. 37: 1007-1013.

22   Price, A.B., Smith, A., Levi, J., Clark, J., Dolby,
      J.M., Stephenson, M.L. and Dunscombe, P.R. 1985,
      Campylobacter pyloridis in peptic ulcer disease:
      pathology, microbiology and scanning electron
      microscopy. J. Clin. Pathol. (in press).

23   Public Health Laboratory Service. 1985.
      Campylobacter III. Proceedings: Third international
      Workshop on Campylobacter infections, A.D. Pearson,
      M.B. Skirrow, H. Lior and B. Rowe (eds.) (in press).

24   Riley, L.W. and Finch, M.W.   1985.   Results of the
      First Year of National Surveillance of campylobacter
      infections in the United States.
      J. Infect. Dis.   151: 956-959.

25   Roop, R.M., Smibert, R.M. and Kreig, N.R.   1984.
      Improved bio-typing schemes for *Campylobacter jejuni*
      and *Campylobacter coli*.
      J. Clin. Microbiol. 20: 990-992.

26   Skirrow, M.B.   1977.   Campylobacter enteritis: a
      'new' disease.   Brit. Med. J.   2: 9-11,

27   Skirrow, M.B. and Benjamin, J.   1980.   1001
      campylobacters: cultural characteristics of
      intestinal campylobacters from man and animals.
      J. Hyg. Camb.   85: 427-442.

28   Steele, T.W., Sangster, N. and Lanser J.A. 1985.
      DNA relatedness and biochemical features of
      Campylobacter spp. isolated in central and South
      Australia.   J. Clin. Microbiol.   22:   71-74.

29   Tauxe, R.V., Patton, C.M., Edmonds, P., Barrett,
      T.J., Brenner, D.J. and Blake, P.A. 1985.   Illness
      associated with *Campylobacter laridis*, a newly
      recognised Campylobacter species.
      J. Clin. Microbiol.   21: 222-225.

30   Totten, P.A., Fennell, C.L., Tenoven, F.C.,
      Wezenberg, J.M., Perine, P.L., Stamm, W.E. and
      Holmes, K.K.   1985.   *Campylobacter cinaedi* (sp.
      nov.) and *Campylobacter fennelliae* (sp. nov.):   two
      new campylobacter species associated with enteric
      disease in homosexual men.   J. Infect. Dis.   151: 131-139.

31   Wenman, W.M., Chai, J., Louie, T.J., Goudreau, C,
      Lior, H., Newell, D.G., Pearson, A.D. and Taylor,
      D.E.   1985.   Antigenic analysis of Campylobacter
      flagella protein and other proteins.
      J. Clin. Microbiol.   21:   108-112.

CHAPTER 6

INTESTINAL SPIROCHETOSIS IN MAN AND OTHER ANIMALS.

Kari Hovind-Hougen

State Veterinary Serum Laboratory, Copenhagen, Denmark.

Contents

Extended abstract

Further reading

Intestinal spirochetosis in man is characterized by a massive infestation of spirochetes in the lumen of the colon and appendix. The spirochetes attach to the epithelial cells at the bases of the microvilli. The epithelial cells appear unaffected in spite of the massive infestation. The only difference between cells with and without attached spirochetes is that the microvilli were shorter and more sparse when spirochetes were present. It has not been possible to obtain any correlation between clinical symptoms and the presence of the intestinal spirochetes. The spirochetes, called *Brachyspira aalborgi*, were originally isolated from rectal biopsies from patients with intestinal spirochetosis. The organisms can be cultivated on trypticase soy agar plates supplemented with 5% calf blood. They grow very slowly and need 2 weeks of incubation to produce small, barely visible colonies. Two kinds of colonies were usually isolated, one was flat, slowly spreading and showed a very weak haemolysis. The other was convex with no detectable haemolysis. Both were colourless. Spirochaetes have been isolated from rectal biopsies and from faeces. Whether or not persons with intestinal spirochetosis produce anti-bodies against the spirochetes they carry is presently unknown.

Intestinal spirochetosis in swine is characterized by a high number of spirochetes present in the colonic lumen as well as in the crypts. The spirochetes have not been seen to attach to epithelial cells. The colonic epithelium is heavily damaged in pigs with swine dysentery and pigs with spirochetal colitis. The tissue disintegrates and sloughed off cells are dispersed in the lumen. Occasionally spirochetes are observed between such disintegrated cells. Alterations of the intestinal epithelial cells were also observed in pigs which were clinically healthy after being fed with strongly haemolytic spirochetes. Examples of these cellular substructural changes were such as short and sparse microvilli and swollen and burst mitochondria together with dilated endoplasmic reticulum. The spiro-chaetes which cause swine dysentery, *Treponema hyodysenteriae*, can also be cultivated on trypticase soy agar plates supplemented with 5% calf blood. They form small colour-less colonies and are strongly haemolytic; the haemolysis is detectable after two days of incubation whereas the colonies are first visible after three to four days of growth. The strongly haemolytic spirochetes vary in lengths, wavelengths and number of flagella. They are morphologically distinguishable from most of the spirochetes which show haemolysis of medium intensity. These latter organisms are generally thinner than the former and possess a distinct substructure at the tip of the cells. The morphology of the weakly haemolytic spirochetes, *Treponema innocens*, is rather similar to that of the strongly haemolytic ones. By morphological criteria the cells of swine spirochetes here mentioned are much more similar to those of the genus *Borrelia* than to those of *Treponema*, and should, in my opinion, be reclassified.

Further Reading

1   Hovind-Hougen, K., Birch-Andersen, A.,Henrik-Nielsen,
     R., Orholm, M., Pedersen, J.O., Teglbjaerg P.S. and
     E.H. Thaysen, E.H.   1982. Intestinal spirochetosis:
     Morphological characterization and cultivation of the
     spirochete *Brachyspira aalborgi* gen. nov., sp.   nov.
     J. Clin. Microbiol.   16: 1127-1136,

2   Henrik-Nielsen, R., Orholm, M., Pedersen, J.O.,
     Hovind-Hougen, K., Teglbjaerg, P.S. and Thaysen, E.H.
     1983.   Colorectal spirochetosis: Clinical
     significance of the ingestation.
     Gastroenterology   85: 62-67.

3   Henrik-Nielsen, R., Lundbeck, F.A., Teglbjaerg, P.S.,
     Ginnerup, P. and Hovind-Hougen, K.   1985.   Intestinal
     spirochetosis of the vermiform appendix.
     Gastroenterology   88: 971-977.

CHAPTER 7

ANAEROBES AND INFLAMMATORY BOWEL DISEASE.

Michael J. Hudson

Bacterial Metabolism Research Laboratory, PHLS Centre for
Applied Microbiological Research, Porton Down, Wiltshire,
SP4 OJG, UK.

Contents

Abstract

Introduction

Antibacterial chemotherapy of IBD

Faecal flora studies

Mucosa-associated flora studies

Immunological studies

Anaerobes and cancer in IBD

An animal model of Ulcerative colitis

Summary and conclusions

References

ABSTRACT

The inflammatory bowel diseases are of unknown aetiology and many aspects of their pathogenesis remain unclear. The clinical usefulness of antimicrobial agents, micro-biological and immunological studies all tend to implicate the gut microflora in the maintenance of IBD, and obligate anaerobes in particular. Bacteria may also be implicated in the development of cancer in IBD.

INTRODUCTION

The idiopathic or non-specific inflammatory bowel diseases (IBD) include ulcerative colitis (UC), proctitis and Crohn's disease (CD). Although the majority of cases are relatively easily differentiated, the inflammatory bowel diseases share many clinical and patho-physiogical features which suggests they may comprise a continuous spectrum of disease (8). A unifying hypothesis for the aetiology and pathogenesis of IBD supposes that an initial insult to the integrity of the mucosal barrier allows antigenic material (microbial, dietary, etc.) normally confined to the lumen to stimulate the local immune system and initiate an immune response; subsequent damage to the mucosa mediated by the inflammatory response, specific autoimmune phenomena, immune-complexes, etc., would result in further immune stimulation and the establishment of chronic disease, susceptible to exacerbation by further transient insult (infection, diet, stress, ischaemia, etc.). The nature of the resultant IBD would depend upon factors such as the site and nature of the immune response, antigens involved and genetic predisposition.

Indirect evidence for a role for microbes in IBD comes from observations of epidemiology, familial clustering, diet associations, etc. Animal transmission studies have incriminated a filterable initiating agent (<0.2 microns) and a variety of candidate organisms (viruses, mycoplasma, chlamydia, cell-wall deficient bacteria) have been isolated by a different groups (see 6) but none have sought CWD or filterable anaerobes (mycoplasmas, treponemas, etc.). Collaborative sudies would help to clarify the significance of these possible aetiological agents.

Evidence for the involvement of anaerobic gut bacteria in the maintenance of IBD comes from similarities of enteric and systemic complications seen in IBD and intestinal bypass surgery (IB), the efficacy of antimicrobial therapy and immunological and microbiological studies.

This paper deals with some of the evidence indicating a role for intestinal anaerobes in IBD, some new approaches to the study of the mechanisms involved and a consideration of a bacterial aetiology for cancer in IBD.

ANTIBACTERIAL CHEMOTHERAPY OF IBD

Recent reports of the usefulness of prolonged treatment with broad-spectrum anti-microbial agents (13) and of metronidazole in particular (19) in the treatmnet of CD have rekindled clinical interest in the role of gut bacteria in IBD. Of course, sulphasalazine (salicyl-azosulphapyridine) has long been used in the treatment of acute IBD and maintenance of remission in UC. This drug is split by gut bacterial azoreductase to sulphapyridine and 5-aminosalicylic acid. Sulphasalazine and the latter aspirin-like moiety are potent inhibitors of prostaglandin synthesis, and this is considered to be the mode of action. Recent studies, however, have confirmed an antibacterial effect, attributable to the sulphapyridine moiety, on the anaerobic faecal flora, particularly *Bacteroides* sp. (9,11,23).

Several clinical trials have confirmed the observations of Ursing and Kamme (19) of the efficacy of metronidazole in the treatment of CD whatever the site of disease (see 7). Krook and colleagues (9,10) showed that clinical improvement during metronidazole treatment of CD was paralleled by a reduction in faecal *Bacteroides* sp. and a concommitant rise in faecal streptococci. We observed these same changes in both the faecal flora and rectal mucosa-associated flora of CD patients taking a combination of metronidazole with cotrimoxazole (7).

The use of oral vancomycin as an adjunct treatmnet of acute UC in the absence of *Clostridium difficile* or its toxin (2) requires confirmation and studies of its effect on the microflora.

FAECAL FLORA STUDIES

Comparison of feacal flora studies is difficult due to widely differing techniques of ensuring anaerobiosis, culture media, selection and identification, etc. Past workers reported disparate results (6,8) but even recent studies using appropriate methods have found no consistent differences between IBD and controls (11) or increased anaerobic bacteria attributed to *B. vulgatus* and to the "*B. fragilis* group" organisms (17,20) or Gram-positive coccoid rods (20). No particular *B. vulgatus* serogroup has been found to be associated with IBD (14). A major difference between IBD patients appears to be non-specific reduction in the flora by 1 or 2 orders of magnitude in patients with acute disease ($10^{8.5}$ to $10^{9.5}$/g) compared with healthy control values ($10^{10.5}$/g), probably as a non-specific effect of diarrhoea and mucus, etc. (7,11,20).

Given the difficulties in matching patient groups, past treatments, etc. in faecal flora studies of IBD, follow-up studies of individual patients might be expected to yield more consistent data.

That acute exacerbation of IBD is due to *C. difficile* overgrowth and toxin elaboration has not been confirmed in prospective studies. However, frequent exposure to anti-microbial agents and hospital environments does put IBD patients into a higher risk category, as they are for enteric infections in general, and the possibility of *C. difficile* superinfection should always be considered in severe relapse after antibiotic use.

Table 1. Mucosa-associated flora of resected colorectal tissue.

	(data from 16)		(Hudson and Hill) unpublished)		
	Control	Crohn's disease	Control	Ulcerative colitis	Toxic UC
Obligate anaerobes					
Total	6.1	6.6	6.4	6.2	5.8
Range	3.1–6.3	3.4–7.4	4.9–7.2	5.8–6.9	4.8–6.1
Bacteroides	64%	61%	72%	80%	72%
Bifidobacterium	9%	14%	12%	12%	8%
Clostridium	4%	6%	<1%	2%	5%
Facultative anaerobes					
Total	5.6	6.7	6.2	5.9	5.7
Range	4.1–6.0	1.7–7.6	4.5–7.0	2.3–6.8	5.1–6.0
Enterobacteria	45%	59%	40%	42%	78%
Streptococci	40%	32%	42%	56%	15%

MUCOSA-ASSOCIATED FLORA STUDIES

The mucosa-associated flora (MAF) has a greater pathogenic potential for involvement in IBD than the lumen flora, and may also act as a protective barrier to invasive organisms. It may be studied using whole-thickness surgically resected bowel, endoscopic or sigmoidscopic mucosal biopsy. Peach and Tabaqchali (16) dexribed the mucosa-associated flora (MAF) of resected small and large intestine from patients with Crohn's disease. The ratio of anaerobic to aerobic bacteria was reduced to near unity but the flora was qualitatively similar to the faecal flora. Table 1 shows the data for the colorectal MAF in Crohn's disease together with comparable data for patients with ulcerative colitis.

In neither study was the MAF found to vary markedly along the colorectum, although the flora associated with small bowel mucosa appeared less dense in both resected and colonoscopy specimens (16). The MAF of recto-sigmoid tissue taken at routine sigmoidoscopy of patients with either UC or CD has an anaerobe/aerobe ratio of about 40 to 1 compared to 5 to 1 for comparable resected tissue, and may be sampled periodically during the course of the disease or treatment. We have shown that treatment of CD with a combination of metronidazole and cotrimoxazole for two weeks results in significant reduction of anaerobes, of the "*B. fragilis* group" in particular, and of enterobacteria, whereas numbers of the latter were unchanged in faeces (7). Differential sensitivity *in vivo* of MAF and faecal flora to antimicrobial agnets has also been observed for phthalyl-sulphathiazole (16). We are currently compiling a library of rectal biopsy specimens taken at routine IBD follow-up in order to study changes in the MAF of each patient with respect to disease activity.

We have also examined isolates of the MAF and faecal flora from patients with untreated active IBD and controls for IgA$_1$-and sIgA specific protease activity (1). It appears that survival on the mucosa is not dependent on evasion of the local IgA system, since few isolates of either faecal or MAF expressed this property.

IMMUNOLOGICAL STUDIES

Elevated serum antibodies directed against "*B. fragilis* group" organisms have been reported in both UC and CD patients by a variety of assays (6,7). Serum agglutins against four Gram-positive coccoid rods (two *Eubacterium* spp., one *Peptostreptococcus* sp. and one *Coprococcus* sp.) are found significantly more frequently in patients with IBD, particularly CD, than in healthy or diseased controls (21). International collaborative studies using this assay (Table 2) suggest that, whatever its pathogenic significance, it has considerable potential as a screening test for the diagnosis of Crohn's disease (22). Abnormal levels of serum antibody against numerically dominant components of the normal intestinal microflora may merely reflect a damaged mucosa.

Table 2. Serologic response to anaerobic Gram-positive coccoid rods

	Positive result %	95% Confid. limits %	Median %	Range %
Crohn's disease	59	53–64	57	35–83
Ulcerative colitis	29	24–34	30	11–63
Healthy control	8	5–12	10	0–33
Disease control	8	4–16	0	0–24

(data from 22; 937 sera from 17 centres in 14 countries)

Colorectal mucosal immunoglobulins of patients with UC are primarily directed against anerobic bacteria whereas serum activity, if any, is directed against aerobes (12). Similarly, immunoblotting studies suggest mucosal rather than serum immunoglobulins are directed against predominant faecal antigens, especially in colitics (4). Such studies designed to identify the antigens involved in the stimulation of the mucosal immunocytes and/or immune-complex formulation are of crucial importance to our understanding of the pathogenesis of inflammatory bowel disease.

ANAEROBES AND CANCER IN IBD

Ulcerative colitis (and probably CD) with toal bowel involvement, early onset and duration of more than 10 years is a premalignant condition (3), necessitating regular follow-up studies of high-risk patients to detect early dysplastic changes in the colorectal epithelium. Faecal carriage of bile acid nuclear dehydrogenating clostridia (NDC) implicated in the aetiology of colorectal cancer (5) has been studied in 92 patients with chronic total ulcerative colitis. Subsequent development of severe dysplasia or carcinoma (8/92) was confined to those patients (22/92) with high faecal bile acid concentrations (>10 mg/g), and of those with high faecal bile acids and dysplasia, 5/8 (63%) were NDC positive compared to 3/14 (21%) NDC negative. These results suggest that faecal bile acids are correlated with the risk of dysplasia in UC and thus tend to support the hypothesis that faecal bile acids are metabolised to genotoxic species or act as promotors.

AN ANIMAL MODEL OF ULCERATIVE COLITIS

Guinea-pigs, rabbits or mice fed degraded carrageenan

develop a chronic ulcerative colitis and caecitis which acn be used to model the human disease. Ulceration is not produced ·in germ-free animals nor in conventional animals given prior treatment with either metronidazole or cotrimoxazole and barrier isolation, indicating the importance of an intact intestinal flora and a role for enterobacteria and/or anaerobes in the formation of ulcers. Onderdonk and colleagues (15) found that carageenan-induced ulceration was dependent upon the presence of *B. vulgatus* as part of that flora, and that the severity of the lesions could be enhanced by both feeding and parenteral immunisation with homologous *B. vulgatus*. Significantly, some inflammatory changes were seen in the intestines of immunised animals not fed carageenan and control studies with *B. fragilis* confirmed the specificity of the model for *B. vulgatus*.

Further refinement of the model should permit the elucidation of the specific nature of the interaction of intestinal bacteria (particularly *B. vulgatus*) and the immune system in the maintenance of chronic colitis.

SUMMARY AND CONCLUSIONS

The aetiology and many aspects of the pathogenesis of IBD remain uncertain. The changes in intestinal florae, abnormal immune response, etc. may all be epiphenomena to some other mechanism of pathogenesis such as altered enterocyte physiology, mucin or eicosanoid synthesis. Taken together, the evidence suggests that *B. vulgatus* is worthy of consideration as the antigenic stimulus which incites the local immune response in IBD, together with the anaerobic Gram-positive coccoid rods. There is a need to study both mucosal antibodies and the MAF along the gut, and of healthy and diseased tissues, with particular reference to the microecology of bacteroides and Gram-positive coccoid rods to clarify their relative significance in IBD; given the diversity of species present in the gut, a closer examination of potentially cytopathic bacterial metabolites (volatile amines, phenols etc.) would seem warranted in the search for those factors eliciting inflammatory response. Of course, preliminary observations of an association of clostridia, faecal bile acids and subsequent development of dysplasia and cancer in IBD requires a larger prospective cohort study to evaluate the use of these assays to screen for those patients at high risk of dysplasia and cancer in IBD.

References

1   Barr, G.D., Hudson, M.J, Priddle, J.D. and Jewell,
     D.P. 1986. Colonic proteases to IgA₁ and sIgA in
     patients with ulcerative colitis - a negative
     study.Gut. (In press).

2   Dickinson, R.J., O'Connor, H.J., Pinder, I.,
     Hamilton, I., Johnston, D. and Axon, A.T.R. 1985.
     Double blind controlled trial of oral vancomycin as
     adjunctive treatment in acute exacerbations of
     idiopathic colitis. Gut 26: 1380-1384.

3   Dobbins, W.O. III. 1984. Dysplasia and malignancy
     in inflammatory bowel disease.
     Ann. Rev. Med. 35: 33-48.

4   Folkersen, J., Sofeldt, S. and Svehag, S-E. 1985.
     Application of electroblotting techniques to studies
     of the intestinal antibody response to extractable
     fecal antigens. Scand. J. Gastroent. 20: 247-253.

5   Hill,M.J. 1975. Bacteria and large bowel cancer.
     Cancer. 36: 2387-2400.

6   Hill, M.J. and Hudson, M.J. 1982. Intestinal
     microflora in inflammatory bowel disease. In: T.
     Shiratori and H. Nakano (eds). Inflammatory bowel
     disease. University of Tokyo Press. pp3-22.

7   Hudson M.J., Hill, M.J., Elliot, P.R., Berghouse,
     L.M., Burnham, W.R. and Lennard-Jones, J.E. 1984.
     The microbial flora of the rectal mucosa and faeces
     of patients with Crohn's disease before and during
     antimicrobial chemotherapy.
     J. Med. Microbiol. 18: 335-345.

8   Kirsner, J.B. and Shorter, R.G. 1982. Recent
     developments in inflammatory bowel disease. N. Engl.
     J. Med. 306: 837-848.

9   Krook, A., Danielsson, D., Kjellander, J and
     Jarnerot, G. 1981. The effect of metronidazole and
     sulfasalazine on the faecal flora in patients with
     Crohn's disease. Scand. J. Gastroent. 16: 183-192.

10   Krook,A., Jarnerot, G. and Danielsson, D. 1981.
     Clinical effect of   metronidazole and
     sulfasalazine on Crohn's disease in relation to
     changes in the faecal flora. Scand. J. Gastroent.
     16: 569-575.

11   Mitsuoka, T. and Benno, Y. 1984. Bacterial species of
     intestinal microflora of patients with inflammatory
     bowel disease. In.: T. Shiratori and H. Nakano
     (eds.). Inflammatory bowel disease. Univ. of Tokyo
     Press. pp35-42.

12   Monteiro, E., Fossey, J., Shiner, M. Drasar, B.S. and
     Allison, A.C. 1971. Antibacterial antibodies in
     rectal and colonic mucosa in ulcerative colitis.
     Lancet. i:249-251.

13   Moss, A.A., Carbone,J.V. and Kressel,H.Y. 1978.
      Radiologic and clinical assessment of broad spectrum
      antibiotic therapy in Crohn's disease.
      Am. J. Roentgenol. 131: 787-790.

14   Okamura, N., Miyazaki, K., Chida, T., Niwayama, K.,
      Nakaya, R., Benno, Y. and Mitsuoka, T. 1985.
      Serogrouping of *Bacteroides vulgatus* by the
      agglutination test. J. Clin Microbiol. 22: 56-61.

15   Onderdonk, A.B., Cisneros, R.L. and Bronson, R.T.
      1983. Enhancement of experimental ulcerative colitis
      by immunization with *Bacteroides vulgatus.*
      Infect. Immun. 42:783-788.

16   Peach, S.L. and Tabaqchali, S. 1982. Mucosa-
      associated flora of the human gastrointestinal tract
      in health and disease.
      Eur. J. Chemother. Antibiotic. 2: 41-50.

17   Ruseler van Embden , J.G.H. and Both-Patoir, H.C.
      1983. Anaerobic Gram-negative faecal flora in
      patients with Crohn's disease and healthy subjects.
      Anton. van Leeuwen. 49: 123-132.

18   Thayer, W.R. and Kirsner, J.B. 1980. Enteric and
      extra-enteric complications of intestinal bypass and
      inflammatory bowel disease. Are there some clues?
      Gastroent. 78: 1097-1100.

19   Ursing, B. and Kamme, C. 1975. Metronidazole for
      Crohn's disease. Lancet. i: 775-777.

20   Wensinck, F., Custer-van Lieshout, L.M.C.,
      Poppelaars-Kustermans, P.A.J. and Schroder,A.M. 1981.
      The faecal flora of patients with Crohn's disease.
      J.Hyg., Camb. 87: 1-12.

21   Wensinck, F. and Van der Nerwe, J.P. 1981. Serum
      agglutins to *Eubacterium* and *Peptostreptococcus*
      species in Crohn's and other diseases.
      J. Hyg., Camb. 87: 13-24.

22.   Wensinck, F. Van der Merwe, J.P. and Mayberry, J.F.
      1983. An international study of agglutins to
      Eubacterium, *Peptostreptococcus* and *Coprococcus*
      species in Crohn's disease and control subjects.
      Digestion. 27: 63-69.

23.   West, B., Lendrum, R. Hill, M.J. and Walker, G.
      1974. Effects of sulphasalazine (Salazopyrin) on
      faecal flora in patients with inflammatory bowel
      disease. Gut. 15: 960-965.

SECTION 3. ANTIBIOTICS AND ANAEROBES

Co-chairman of session : Professor I. Phillips

Professor C. E. Nord

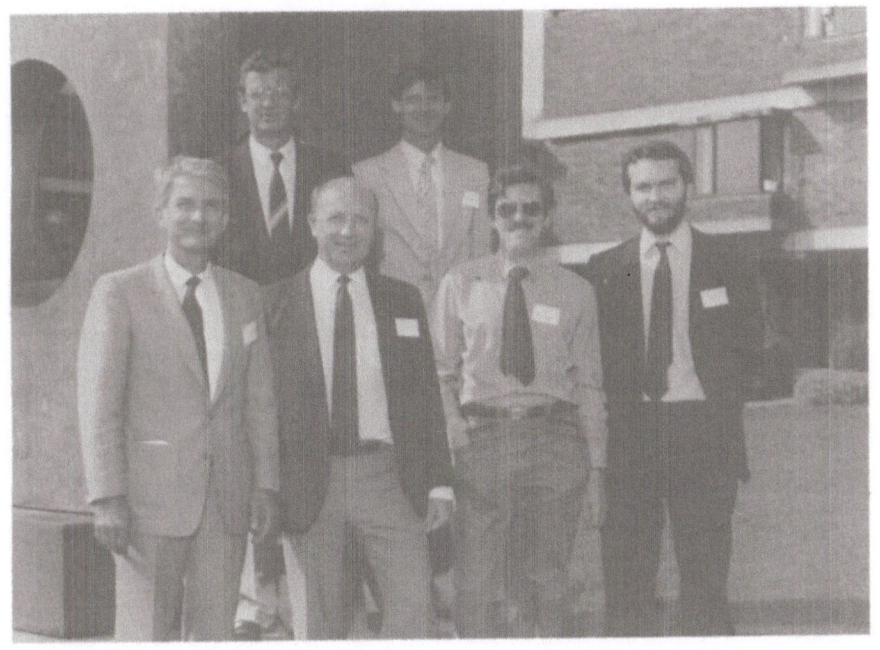

From left to right :-

Back row : C.E. Nord, C.G. Gemmell

Front row : D. van der Waaij, I. Phillips, C.S. Stewart and A. Eley.

CHAPTER 8

NEWER ANTIBIOTICS ACTIVE AGAINST *BACTEROIDES FRAGILIS* : COMPARISON WITH OLDER AGENTS

Adrian Eley and David Greenwood

Department of Microbiology and PHLS Laboratory, University Hospital, Queen's Medical Centre, Nottingham, NG7 2UH, UK.

Contents

Abstract

Introduction

Materials and methods

      Bacterial strain

      Antibiotics

      Culture medium

      Antibiotic titrations

      Turbidimetric studies

      Viable counts

      Microscopy

Results

      Anitibiotic titrations

      Turbidimetric experiments

      Inoculum effects

      Comparative bactericidal activity

      Relationship of activity and achievable blood levels

      Activity on stationary phase cultures

Discussion

References

NEWER ANTIBIOTICS ACTIVE AGAINST *BACTEROIDES FRAGILIS* : COMPARISON WITH OLDER AGENTS

Adrian Eley and David Greenwood

ABSTRACT

The activity of eleven antibiotics against a high inoculum (*ca* 10^8 cfu./ml) of *Bacteroides fragilis* was examined in an anaerobic turbidimeter which allowed the removal of samples during the course of the experiment for the parallel investigation of bactericidal activity and morphological effects. When comparative bacteriostatic and bactericidal activities were related to achievable blood levels, imipenem, clindamycin and the combination of benzylpenicillin with clavulanic acid exhibited the highest activity. Surprisingly, fusidic acid also showed good activity. Although metronidazole displayed only moderate bacteriostatic and bactericidal activity in relation to achievable blood levels it was the only agent found to be bactericidal to cultures in the stationary phase of growth, and this may help to explain its excellent activity *in vivo*.

INTRODUCTION

There has been increasing interest shown in anaerobic bacteria during the last few years, due largely to growing recognition of the importance of anaerobic bacteria as significant causes of infections in man. At present there are four classes of antimicrobial agents are advocated for the treatment of anaerobic infections, including those caused by *Bacteroides fragilis*: nitroimidazoles (metronidazole and tinidazole); clindamycin; chloramphenicol; and certain beta-lactam antibiotics (cefoxitin, latamoxef, carboxypenicillins, acylureidopenicillins and the combination of amoxycillin and clavulanic acid). Erythromycin has been advocated for the less serious anaerobic infections involving soft tissue, the oral cavity or lung (14), and fusidic acid has quite good anti-anaerobe activity *in vitro* (22). Among investigational compounds presently in clinical trials, the novel beta-lactam antibiotic imipenem (N-formimidoyl thienamycin), and ciprofloxacin, one of the newer quinolone antibiotics, also display useful activity against *B. fragilis* (3,9).

The susceptibility of bacteria to antimicrobial agents is traditionally determined by in-vitro tests with relatively low inocula. However, the validity of these results is open to debate since high inocula (10^7 – 10^9 cfu/ml) are commonly found in infected lesions, including anaerobic abscesses (1). A great deal of information about the comparative response to antibiotics of high and low inocula of bacteria can be obtained by continuous turbidimetric monitoring techniques, especially when performed in parallel with microscopy to observe antibiotic-induced morphological changes, viable counts to assess bactericidal activity, and assays to provide evidence of drug inactivation.

In the present study, these techniques have been used to compare the activities of eleven anti-anaerobe agents against a type culture strain of *B. fragilis*.

MATERIALS AND METHODS

Bacterial strain. *Bacteroides fragilis* NCTC 9344 was used throughout.

Antibiotics. Cefoxitin and imipenem (Merck, Sharp and Dohme Ltd), benzylpenicillin (Glaxo Group Research Ltd), clavulanic acid (Beecham Pharmaceuticals), latamoxef (Eli

Lilly and Co. Ltd), metronidazole (May and Baker Ltd), clindamycin (Upjohn Ltd), erythromycin (Abbott Laboratories Ltd), chloramphenicol (Parke, Davis and Co. Ltd), fusidic acid (Leo Pharmaceutical Products), piperacillin (Lederle Laboratories) and ciprofloxacin (Bayer UK Ltd) were obtained from the manufacturers or as standard pharmaceutical preparations from the hospital pharmacy. Solutions of antibacterial agents were freshly prepared as required. Solutions of ciprofloxacin and chloramphenicol were prepared in sterile distilled water after dissolving weighed powder in a small volume (<1ml) of 1M NaOH and methanol respectively. Imipenem was dissolved in 0.01 1M phosphate buffer (pH 7.0) according to the manufacturer's instructions. Solutions of the remaining compounds were prepared by dissolving weighed powder in sterile distilled water.

The beta-lactamase inhibitor, clavulanic acid, was used at a concentration of 4 mcg/ml in all experiments with benzyl-penicillin.

Culture medium. Brain heart infusion broth supplemented with yeast extract 5 mg/ml, haemin 5 mcg/ml and menadione 1 mcg/ml (BHIS) was used throughout. This medium was previously shown to be the most suitable of several anaerobic culture media for the growth of organisms of the *B. fragilis* group (6). All culture media were pre-reduced by incubation overnight in a mixture of N_2 80% : CO_2 10% and H_2 10%.

Antibiotic titrations. Minimum inhibitory concentrations (MICs) of antibiotics were determined by the broth dilution method. Serial two-fold dilutions of antibiotics were prepared in 1 ml volumes of BHIS and one drop of a 1 in

1000 dilution of an overnight culture of the test organism in BHIS was added to achieve a final inoculum of *ca* 10^4 cfu/ml. Results were read after overnight incubation at 37°C. in an anaerobic jar.

Turbidimetric studies. Bacteria from overnight broth cultures were inoculated into 9 ml volumes of pre-reduced BHIS. Antibiotic was added either when bacterial growth had raised the opacity of the cultures to a level of 30% (*ca* 10^8 cfu/ml) of that obtained with a fully grown broth culture, or when organisms were judged to have reached the early stationary phase (*ca* 10^9 cfu/ml). The tubes were incubated anaerobically in a six channel turbidimeter as described elsewhere (15). In this system, antibiotic can be added during growth, or samples removed for further testing, without disturbing anaerobiosis.

To detect antibiotic breakdown, cultures exposed over-night to antibiotic were centrifuged at 3,000 rpm for 20 min. Supernatant fluids were removed and assayed by a well-diffusion technique with *Staphylococcus aureus* NCTC 6571 or *Escherichia coli* NCTC 10418 as the indicator organism (5). The activity of metronidazole was determined by an anaerobic microbiological assay with *Clostridium sporogenes* as indicator organism (18).

Viable counts. Broth-culture samples removed at appropriate intervals during the course of turbidimetric experiments were examined for viability by the agar droplet method (20). Samples were diluted in serial ten-fold steps in fresh BHIS broth, with a final dilution in BHIS agar (BHIS solidified with 1% agar) by use of the Colworth "Droplette' dispenser (A.J. Seward Ltd, London). Colonies in the agar droplets were counted by use of the illumi-nated magnifier and counter unit incorporated in the

'Droplette' device. Viable counts were expressed as the mean number of cfu/ml in quintuplicate samples of the appropriate dilutions.

<u>Microscopy</u>. Antibiotic-induced morphological changes in bacteria were observed by interference-contrast microscopy of samples taken from turbidimetric experiments 60 min after addition of antibiotic and after overnight (22 hr) incubation.

RESULTS

<u>Antibiotic titrations</u>. Minimum inhibitory concentrations (MICs) of all antibiotics estimated in broth titration with an inoculum of *ca* 10^4 cfu/ml are shown in table 1. Clindamycin displayed the highest activity which was 1064 fold greater than that of cefoxitin, the least active of

Table 1. Activity of eleven antibiotics against *Bacteroides fragilis* NCTC 9344

| Antibacterial agent | Antibacterial activity (mcg/ml) as judged by | | | | |
| | Conventional | <u>Turbidimetric</u> | | <u>Bactericidal effect at**</u> | |
	MIC*	MAC+	MIC+	3h	24h
Metronidazole	0.5	2	>8	4	4
Clindamycin	0.0075	0.06	0.12	0.25	0.25
Erythromycin	1	0.5	2	16	8
Chloramphenicol	1	2	8	32	16
Fusidic acid	1	0.25	4	8	4
Ciprofloxacin	4	4	16	64	16
Cefoxitin	8	4	8	16	16
Piperacillin	2	4	32	32	32
Latamoxef	0.25	2	4	16	4
Imipenem	0.12	0.25	1	1	1
Benzylpenicillin & clavulanic acid	0.12	0.5	1	1	1

MAC = minimum antibacterial concentration (concentration causing a significant deviation from normal growth);
MIC = minimum inhibitory concentration (concentration suppressing growth overnight)
* inoculum = *ca* 10^4 cfu/ml
+ inoculum = *ca* 10^8 cfu/ml
** Bactericidal effect (MBC) defined as 99% killing after 3 h,
                                            99% killing after 24 h.

the antibiotics tested.

Turbidimetric experiments.   The response of *B. fragilis*
NCTC 9344 to antibiotics was observed by continuous turbidimetric monitoring.   Antibiotic was added when bacterial
growth had raised the inoculum to *ca* 10^8 cfu/ml.   Typical
findings obtained are shown in Fig. 1 which illustrates
the response of *B. fragilis* NCTC 9344 to the two most
active drugs, imipenem (Fig. 1a) and clindamycin (Fig. 1b),
typifying the response to beta-lactam and non beta-lactam
compounds respectively.

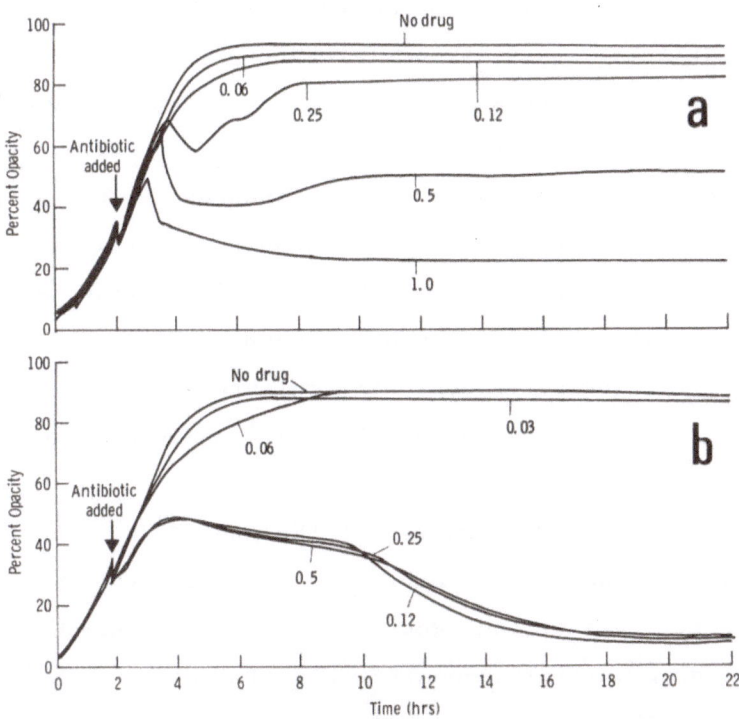

Figure 1.   Continuous opacity records of *Bacteroides fragilis* NCTC
9344.   Imipenem (a) and clindamycin (b) added at arrow to achieve
the concentrations (mcg/ml) shown.

Exposure of the test organism to a beta- lactam drug
typically caused a bacteriolytic effect which occurred
more rapidly as the drug concentration was increased.

Interference contrast microscopy revealed that lysis was accompanied by the formation of large numbers of spheroplasts. However, even the highest drug concentration used failed to reduce the final opacity of the culture to below 20% of that of a fully-grown broth culture although no viable bacteria were detected by sub-culture at the end of the experiment. Microscopy revealed a large quantity of lysed cell debris.

In contrast, when the test organism was exposed to a non beta-lactam drug the opacity of the culture continued to increase normally for approx. 2h after exposure to the drug. During this period no morphological changes were seen by interference contrast microscopy, except with ciprofloxacin which caused filamentation at concentrations above 2 mcg/ml. However, after exposure to the drugs for 8 h the opacities started to fall, eventually reaching levels of <10% of that of a fully grown broth culture at the end of the experiment. When these cultures were examined by light microscopy scanty lysed cell debris was found in all cases except in cultures exposed to ciprofloxacin in which many degenerate filaments were seen.

Bioassay of broth supernates at the end of the experiments revealed no loss of activity of either the beta-lactam or non beta-lactam agents, except metronidazole. With this drug initial concentrations of 4 and 8 mcg/ml became undetectable during overnight incubation.

Inoculum effects. Increasing the inoculum size from ca 10^4 cfu/ml in broth titrations to ca 10^8 cfu/ml in turbidimetric experiments dramatically altered the MICs of the majority of antibiotics; however, the MIC of erythromycin was little changed and that of cefoxitin unaltered (table

1). Low-inoculum MICs were mostly comparable to, or slightly lower than, the minimum antibacterial concentrations (MACs) observed in the turbidimetric experiments. Comparative bactericidal activity. The bactericidal activities of the 11 antibiotics were compared in terms of the concentrations achieving a 99% reduction of the original inoculum within 3hr, or a 99.9% reduction within 24hr (table 1). Clindamycin, imipenem and the benzyl-penicillin/clavulanic acid combination exhibited bactericidal activity at concentrations much lower than those of the other compounds.

In order to compare the rates of killing by the 11 agents, killing curves were constructed from the results of experiments in which *B. fragilis* was exposed to each of the test compounds at a concentration equivalent to four

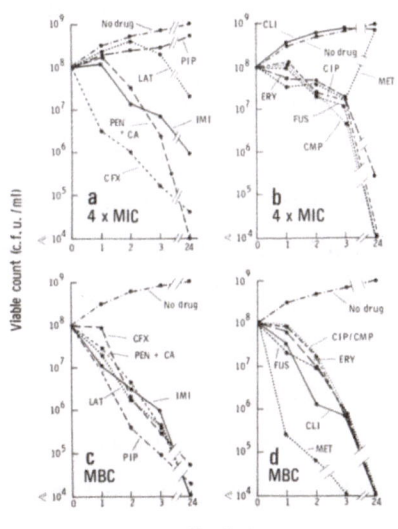

Figure 2. Viable counts of *Bacteroides fragilis* NCTC 9344 when exposed to five beta-lactam agents (a, c) and six non beta-lactam agents (b, d) at concentrations of 4 times the low-inoculum MICs (a,b) and at the minimum bactericidal concentrations (c, d). See table 1 for concentrations used. CFX = cefoxitin; IMI = imipenem; LAT = latamoxef; PEN + CA = benzylpenicillin and clavulanic acid; PIP = piperacillin; CIP = ciprofloxacin; CMP = chloramphenicol; CLI = clindamycin; ERY = erythromycin; FUS = fusidic acid; MET = metronidazole.

times the low inoculum MIC (Fig. 2a, b) and at the minimum
bactericidal concentration (MBC; the concentration achieving
99% killing after 3 h) (Fig. 2c, d). At a concentration
of 4 x MIC, cefoxitin achieved the most rapid bactericidal
effect, whereas piperacillin and clindamycin appeared to
exert no lethal action. After exposure to metronidazole
at a concentration of 4 x MIC, an early fall in viable
count was followed by resumption of growth during overnight incubation. The remaining compounds achieved a slow
bactericidal effect which was maintained on prolonged
exposure.

When the agents were tested at concentrations equivalent
to their respective MBCs (which except in the case of
cefoxitin, were much more than 4 x MIC; see table 1),
piperacillin was marginally the most rapidly bactericidal
of the beta-lactam compounds (Fig. 2c) and metronidazole
was the most rapidly bactericidal of all (Fig.2d).

Relationship of activity to achievable blood levels. The
bacteriostatic and bactericidal activities of the antibiotics tested against a high inoculum (10^8 cfu/ml) were
related to concentrations achievable in blood 30 – 60 min
after administration of maximal safe doses. These levels
were obtained from published data (2,8,10,11,17).

As expected, inhibitory quotients were significantly
higher than the bactericidal quotients of the same drugs
(table 2). However, in general, the comparative activities
of the drugs were similar whether bacteriostatic or
bactericidal criteria were used; in both cases imipenem
and clindamycin were the most active and erythromycin and
ciprofloxacin the least active drugs. Of the other agents
tested, the benzylpenicillin/clavulanic acid combination
displayed good activity, being more active than metronidazole

Table 2.   Relative bacteriostatic and bactericidal activities
of antibiotics against a high inoculum of *B.fragilis* NCTC 9344

Antibacterial agent	Plasma concentration (mcg/ml)	Inhibitory quotient **	Bactericidal quotient *
Imipenem	32	512	32
Clindamycin	8	128	32
Benzylpenicillin (& clavulanic acid)	16	64	16
Fusidic acid	32	64	4
Metronidazole	16	16	4
Latamoxef	32	128	2
Piperacillin	64	8	2
Cefoxitin	32	8	2
Chloramphenicol	16	4	< 1
Erythromycin	4	2	< 1
Ciprofloxacin	4	< 1	< 1

**Achievable blood level Drug concentration inhibiting growth after 3h
 * Achievable blood level Drug concentration achieving 99% killing after
   3 h (MBC)

metronidazole   in   terms   of   inhibitory   and   bactericidal
quotients.   Surprisingly,   fusidic   acid   also   displayed   good
activity   which   was   comparable   to   that   of   metronidazole   in
terms of achievable blood levels.

Activity on stationary phase cultures.   When a stationary
phase   culture   of   *B. fragilis*   NCTC 9344 was   exposed   to
metronidazole at a concentration of 16 mcg/ml for 16 h the
viable count was reduced 100-fold from 1×10^9 to 9.4×10^5 cfu/ml.
None of the other agents caused any reduction in viable count
of stationary phase cultures.

DISCUSSION

    B. fragilis was chosen for this study because it is the most frequently encountered anaerobic pathogen (16). Although a study of only one strain has obvious limitations, the type-culture strain chosen appeared fully typical as judged by antibiotic susceptibility results, and the main findings were confirmed with a fresh clinical isolate of *B. fragilis*. Moreover, the findings where consistent with those reported by others (3,9,21,22,23).

    It has been stated that, ideally, the peak serum concentration of anti-anaerobe drugs should exceed the MIC for the infecting organism by at least fourfold (19). However, in the present study, concentrations of piperacillin and clindamycin equivalent to four times the low inoculum MIC showed little or no activity against dense populations of *B. fragilis*, and the activity of metronidazole was only transient. In terms of bactericidal activity, only cefoxitin was able to achieve a rapidly lethal effect against a dense population of *B. fragilis* at a concentration of 4 x MIC, although most of the other agents tested achieved a marked bactericidal effect on prolonged incubation. More impressive bactericidal activity was achieved when the compounds were tested at the much higher concentrations represented by their respective MBCs, but in the cases of erythromycin, chloramphenicol and ciprofloxacin such concentrations are not readily attainable in the body.

    The relationship between plasma levels and minimum inhibitory concentrations of antibiotics can be expressed as the inhibitory quotient (7), and the concept can clearly be extended to lethal activity. However, in view of variations that may be found in MIC test results, particularly when different inocula are used, it is important that methodology should be standardized if the inhibitory or bactericidal quotients are to have any general validity.

We have elected to use turbidimetric criteria to assess the inhibitory quotient. By this method the inoculum is accurately standardized (because antibiotic is added at a fixed point on the bacterial growth curve) and the dense inoculum involved may be more relevant to clinical reality. Judged in this way, the new carbapenem antibiotic, imipenem, and the lincosamide, clindamycin, appeared to exhibit the highest activity. However, all the agents tested, except erythromycin and ciprofloxacin, exhibited an inhibitory quotient of 4 or more and this may explain the similar efficacy of many anti-anaerobe agents in clinical use (4,12,13).

Nevertheless, only five of the agents tested (imipenem, clindamycin, the benzylpenicillin/clavulanic acid combination, fusidic acid and metronidazole) displayed bactericidal quotients of 4 or more and this may be relevant in those clinical conditions in which a bactericidal effect is judged to be desirable. Furthermore, metronidazole, which is the anti-anaerobe agent presently most favoured in Britain, was the only agent that exhibited bactericidal activity against stationary phase bacteria, a feature which may be of value in certain anaerobic infections.

References

1   Bartlett, J.G., Sullivan-Sigler, N., Louie, T.J. and
    Gorbach, S.L. 1975.   Anaerobes survive in clinical
    specimens despite delayed processing.
    J. Clin. Microbiol. 3: 133-136.

2   Bergeron, M.G., Desaulniers, D., Lessard, C.,
    Lemieux, M., Despres, J-P., Metras, J., Raymond, G.
    and Brochu, G. 1985. Concentrations of fusidic acid,
    cloxacillin and cefamandole in sera and atrial
    appendages of patients undergoing cardiac surgery.
    J. Clin. Microbiol. 27: 928-932.

3   Brown, J.E., Del Bene, V.E. and Collins, C.D. 1981.
    In vitro activity of N-formimidoyl thienamycin,
    moxalactam and other new beta-lactam agents against
    Bacteroides fragilis : Contribution of beta-
    lactamase to resistance.
    Antimicrob. Agents Chemother. 19: 248-252.

4   Collier, J., Colhoun, E.M. and Hill, P.L. 1981. A
    multicentre comparison of clindamycin and
    metronidazole in the treatment of anaerobic
    infections. Scand. J. Infect. Dis., Suppl. 26: 96-100.

5   Eley, A. and Greenwood, D. 1981. *In vitro* activity
    of ceftizoxime against *Bacteroides fragilis* :
    Comparison with benzylpenicillin, cephalothin and
    cefoxitin. Antimicrob. Agents Chemother. 20: 332-335.

6   Eley, A., Greenwood, D. and O'Grady, F. 1985.
    Comparative growth of *Bacteroides* species in various
    anaerobic culture media.
    J. Med. Microbiol. 19: 195-201.

7   Ellner, P.D. and Neu, H.C. 1981. The Inhibitory
    Quotient. J. Amer. Med. Assoc. 246: 1575-1578.

8   Finegold, S.M. 1977. Anaerobic bacteria in human
    disease. Academic Press, Inc., New York.

9   Greenwood, D. Baxter, S., Cowlishaw, A., Eley, A.
    and Slater, G.J. 1984. Antibacterial activity of
    ciprofloxacin in conventional tests and in a model of
    bacterial cystitis.
    Eur. J. Clin. Microbiol. 3: 351-354

10 Hoffler, D., Dalhoff, A., Gau, W., Beerman, D. and
    Michl, A. 1984. Dose and sex independent disposition
    of ciprofloxacin.
    Eur. J. Clin. Microbiol. 3: 363-366.

11 Kirby, B.D., George, W.L., Sutter, V.L., Citron, D.M.
    and Finegold, S.M. 1980. Gram-negative anaerobic
    bacilli : their role in infection and patterns of
    susceptibility to antimicrobial agents. I. Little-
    known *Bacteroides* species.
    Rev. Infect. Dis. 2: 914-951.

12   Klastersky, J., Coppens, L. and Mombelli, G. 1979.
      Anaerobic infection in cancer patients : comparative
      evaluation of clindamycin and cefoxitin.
      Antimicrob. Agents Chemother. 16: 366-371.

13   Ledger, W.J., Moore, D.E., Lewensohn, R.I. and Gee,
      C.L. 1977. A fever index evaluation of
      chloramphenicol or clindamycin in patients with
      serious pelvic infections. Obstet. Gynecol. 50: 523-529.

14   Lewis, R.P., Goldstein, E.J.C., Sutter, V.L. and
      Finegold, S.M. 1978. Erythromycin therapy of
      anaerobic infections. In: Current Chemotherapy. :
      American Society for Microbiology, Washington, D.C.
      p. 653-655.

15   O'Grady, F. and Eley, A. 1983. Continuous opacity
      monitoring of the growth of bacteria under strict
      anaerobic conditions.
      J. Clin. Pathol. 36: 1228-1232.

16   Olsson, B., Dornbusch, K. and Nord, C.E. 1977.
      Susceptibility to beta-lactam antibiotics and
      production of beta-lactamase in *Bacteroides fragilis*.
      Med. Microbiol and Immunol. 163: 183-194.

17   Reeves D S   Holt H A   Bywater M J. and Bidwell
      J.L. 1982.   Comparative activity *in vitro* of
      piperacillin.   J. Antimicrob. Chemother. 9: Suppl B, 59-74.

18   Salem, A., Parnell, M.J. and Jackson, D.D. 1978.
      Metronidazole. In : D.S. Reeves., I. Phillips., J.D.
      Williams and R. Wise (ed.).   Laboratory methods in
      antimicrobial chemotherapy.   Churchill Livingstone,
      Edinburgh.

19   Selkon, J.B. 1981. The need and choice of
      chemotherapy for anaerobic infections.
      Scand. J. Infect. Dis. Suppl. 26: 19-23.

20   Sharpe, A.N. and Kilsby, D.C. 1971. A rapid
      inexpensive bacterial count technique using agar
      droplets. J. Appl. Bact. 34: 435-440.

21   Soriano, F., Ponte, M.C. and Gaspar, M.C. 1982.   The
      in vitro response of *Bacteroides fragilis* to
      moxalactam, cefotaxime, cefmetazole, josamycin and
      erythromycin. J. Clin. Pathol. 35: 1166- 1167.

22   Stirling, J. and Goodwin, S. 1977. Susceptibility of
      Bacteroides fragilis to fusidic acid.
      J. Antimicrob. Chemother. 3: 522-523.

23   Wise R. 1977. Clavulanic acid and susceptibility of
      Bacteroides fragilis to penicillin.   Lancet ii : 145.

CHAPTER 9

INTERACTION OF ANTIBIOTICS, ANAEROBIC BACTERIA AND HOST DEFENCES

Curtis G. Gemmell,

Department of Bacteriology, University of Glasgow
Medical School, Royal Infirmary, Glasgow, UK.

Contents

Abstract

Review

Introduction

References

ABSTRACT

Much of our knowledge of the opsonic requirements of anaerobic bacteria has been developed from the study of various aerobic bacteria. In particular Gram—positive bacterial activate the alternate complement cascade in the absence of any specific antibody, whereas Gram—negative species activate the classical complement cascade usually in the presence of specific antibody. However a combination of both pathways has been described for members of the genus *Bacteroides*. The presence of capsular polysaccharide on the cell surface is recognised as being important in this activation process which may or may not lead to efficient phagocytic ingestion and killing of the bacteria by polymorphonuclear leukocytes (PMNL).

Several antibiotics are concentrated within PMNL but only one drug with activity against anaerobes, clindamycin, can be concentrated up to 40—fold within the phagosome of the PMNL and remain biologically active therein. Alternatively some antibiotics at low concentrations (especially concentrations below the MIC's) have been shown to modify the introduction of various bacteria with PMNL. Again clindamycin has been shown to repress polysaccharide capsule biosynthesis in *Bacteroides fragilis*, and by so doing, to enhance opsonophagocytosis. In contrast, other antibiotics including penicillin and cefoxitin, cause filamentation, increase capsule formation and reduce opsonophagocytosis in the same experimental situation. The significance of these findings *in vivo* in the treatment of the anaerobic abscess remains to be seen.

REVIEW

The susceptibility of *Bacteroides* species to phagocytic ingestion and killing by polymorphonuclear leukocytes (PMNL) and peritoneal macrophages is likely to determine the outcome of the host—parasite interaction within the anaerobic abscess. Some variation in the susceptibility of different strains of *B. fragilis* to phagocytosis has been attributed to the presence or absence of a polysaccharide capsule (13,16). Growth *in vivo* has been shown to enhance the production of the capsule (14) but serial subculture *in vitro* reduced the production of capsulate cells. Impaired phagocytosis of the *in vivo* passaged bacteroides cells was demonstrated (18).

However, *B. fragilis* is not the only member of the genus capable of elaborating a capsule composed of an acidic polyanionic polysaccharide (12); *B. distasonis*, *B. thetaiotaomicron*, and *B. vulgatus* can each synthesize different amounts of this exopolymer (2). Studies of the susceptibility of selected strains to serum opsonization have demonstrated the participation of immunoglobulin and the alternative complement pathway (1), and the classical pathway of complement activation (19). However activation of the classical and/or alternate pathways was not related to the presence or absence of the capsule (2). The concentration of normal human serum required to facilitate maximal opsonization ranged from 5-20% but a few strains required up to 80% serum before opsonophagocytosis occurred. These strains carried increased amounts of polysaccharide on their surface. The opsonic requirements of *B. fragilis* are summarised in table 1. Antibody (IgG) as well as complement was essential for the successful opsonophagocytosis of *B. fragilis* in experimentally infected mice (4).

Table 1. Features of serum opsonisation of *Bacteroides fragilis*

ACTIVATION OF CLASSICAL C PATHWAY – ANTIBACTERIAL ANTIBODY
ACTIVATION OF ALTERNATE C PATHWAY – LIPOPOLYSACCHARIDE
C3 REDISTRIBUTION ON CELL SURFACE – NATURAL ANTIBODY

Serum from mice which survived infection with *B. fragilis* proved to be a better opsonic source than normal mouse serum. Analysis of the *in vitro* killing of *B. fragilis* by peritoneal macrophages showed that optimal killing occurred in the presence of immune serum although normal serum could promote phagocytic killing to an intermediate degree.

The efficacy of phagocytic killing of anaerobic bacteria might be enhanced in two ways. For example some antibiotics can penetrate the membrane of the PMNL and can be concentrated therein (10,15). Prominent amongst these are ciprofloxacin, clindamycin, erythromycin, fusidic acid and rifampicin. However none of these drugs has been used to examine the phagocytosis of *Bacteroides* spp. by PMNL *in vitro*, although there is evidence that enhanced killing of staphylococci can occur in the presence of rifampicin (3). Furthermore, exposure of bacteria to sub-inhibitory concentrations of various antibiotics has been recognised to enhance their susceptibility to opsonophagocytosis (7,17). Surface features (eg. M protein on *Streptococcus pyogenes* and protein A on *Staphylococcus aureus*) were lost during growth in the presence of clindamycin or fusidic acid respectively and potentiation of serum complement-mediated opsonization occurred (5,8).

Primarily because clindamycin is clinically effective against anaerobic infections, a few studies have been directed at the interaction of antibiotic-exposed *B. fragilis* with phagocytic cells *in vitro* (6,11,20). Exposure to clindamycin (1/2 MIC) during growth anaerobically had no effect on cellular morphology. However the degree of encapsulation was reduced (q). In contrast, similar treatment with sub-MIC levels of cefoxitin and penicillin had marked effects on cell morphology, the bacteria becoming long and filamentous. Cefoxitin treatment also resulted in a high percentage of filaments with larger than normal capsules.

When the clindamycin-grown *B. fragilis* cells were opsonized in normal human serum (lacking specific antibody) there was less activation of complement but greater susceptibility to ingestion by PMNL *in vitro* (Table 2). Almost twice as much complement was consumed by the untreated organisms as by those grown in the presence of 1/2 MIC of clindamycin. Transmission electron microscopy revealed capsular polysaccharide on the surface of the bacteroides cells grown in the absence of clindamycin but little or none on the surface of the cells grown in its presence of clindamycin (6). Other changes in the ultrastructure of the cell might take place.

Table 2. Phagocytic uptake of *Bacteroides fragilis* grown in the presence or absence of clindamycin: effect of serum opsonization

Drug treatment	% uptake* by PMN after opsonization in		
	10% serum	20% serum	50% serum
none	26.5	56.4	58.1
1/2 MIC	31.4	69.1	68.5
1/4 MIC	23.2	50.7	55.1
1/8 MIC	21.7	48.2	45.9

* mean of three separate experiments

Modification of the bacteroides cell surface is likely to enhance the adherence of the bacteria to the PMNL surface *via* the receptors for C3b and a subsequent increase in numbers of intracellular bacteria. Confirmatory evidence can be obtained by following the generation of luminol-enhanced chemiluminescence (CL) by PMNL when presented with opsonized bacteroides cells. A typical experiment is illustrated in table 3. Clindamycin-exposed *B. fragilis* cells generated a higher CL response than that induced by cells grown in the absence of any drug. As well as suggesting that increased numbers of bacteroides cells were being ingested by the PMNL it is possible that the biochemical activity of the cell, namely superoxide production, was also being potentiated by the presence of drug-damaged bacteria. The rate at which the intracellular bacteria were killed was also accelerated. There was more than a 1 log decrease in cell numbers when clindamycin-grown *B. fragilis* were allowed to interact with PMNL for 1 h. A much smaller decrease in cell numbers was seen when untreated *B. fragilis* was incubated with PMNL (6). Clindamycin treatment *per se* did not kill the bacteria.

Table 3.   Chemiluminescence of human PMN exposed to clindamycin-damaged *Bacteroides fragilis* cells

Drug treatment	Peak height of chemiluminescence (x10^3)*
none	26.4
1/2 MIC	42.9
1/4 MIC	37.4
1/8 MIC	29.2

* measured as counts per second with an automated luminometer (Packard Instruments Ltd., Caversham, England

Another study (11) addressed the same problem but from a slightly different angle. Bacteroides cells were exposed to various concentrations of clindamycin for 2 h. before their interaction with PMNL and human serum. Even under the limitations of such exposure to the drug, some alteration, although transient, was apparent in the susceptibility of the bacteria to opsonophagocytosis (table 4). Some differences in efficacy of phagocytic killing were apparent after 30 min but not after 60 min. Somewhat conflicting results have been reported (20) when different methods have been used to measure phagocytosis.

Table 4. Effect of exposure of *B. fragilis* cells to clindamycin on their ubsequent susceptibility to phagocytosis

Drug Exposure mg/L	% *B.fragilis* phagocytosed	
	After 30 min	After 60 min
none	0.3 ± 0.3	53.8 ± 3.7
0.004 (1/12 MIC)	3.7 ± 2.6	14.5 ± 11.7
0.01 (1/5 MIC)	21.4 ± 7.6	45.4 ± 2.5
0.02 (2/5 MIC)	8.8 ± 0.6	34.0 ± 6.9

Modified from Howard and Soucy (11)

We shall have to await further investigations to decide whether the host-defense system through the activities of PMNL can distinguish between bacteroides cells exposed to various antibiotics such that potentiation of susceptibility to phagocytosis occurs. It may be that the outcome of the bacteroides-phagocytic cell-antibiotic interaction may be somewhat artificial in these *in vitro* experiments with no counterpart in the anaerobic abscess *in vivo*. Nevertheless comparison of the various antibiotics with biological activity against anaerobic bacteria in the manner described may answer some questions regarding their clinical efficacy. Preliminary studies with other drugs has provided some of the answers (table 5).

Table 5. Antibiotics, PMNL and *Bacteroides fragilis*

Drug	Activity *in vitro*
Cefoxitin	No effect on phagocytosis
Ciprofloxacin	No effect on phagocytosis
Clindamycin	Stimulation of phagocytosis
Metronidazole	No effect on phagocytosis

References

1   Bjornson, A.B. and Bjornson, H.S. 1978. Participation of immunoglobulin and the alternative complement pathway in opsonization of *Bacteroides fragilis* and *Bacteroides thetaiotoamicron*. J. Infect. Dis. 138: 351-358.

2   Bjornson, A.B., Bjornson, H.S., Ashraf, M. and Lang, T.J. 1983. Quantitative variability in requirements for opsonization of strains within the *Bacteroides fragilis* group. J. Infect. Dis. 148: 667-675.

3   Easmon, C.S.F. 1979. The effect of antibiotics on the intracellular survival of *Staphylococcus aureus in vitro*. Brit. J. Exp. Path. 60: 24-28.

4   Ellis, T.M. and Barrett, J.T. 1952. Characterisation of opsonins for *Bacteroides fragilis* in immune sera collected from experimentally infected mice. Infect. Immun. 35: 929-936.

5   Gemmell, C.G. and O'Dowd, A. 1983. Regulation of protein A biosynthesis in *Staphylococcus aureus* by certain antibiotics: its effect on phagocytosis by leukocytes. J. Antimicrob. Chemother. 12: 587-597.

6   Gemmell, C.G., Peterson, P.K, Schmelling D., Mathews, J. and Quie, P.G. 1983. Antibiotic-induced modification of *Bacteroides fragilis* and its susceptibility to phagocytosis by human polymorphonuclear leukocytes. Eur. J. Clin. Microbiol. 2: 327-334.

7   Gemmell, C.G., Peterson,P.K., Schmelling D., Kim, K., Mathews, J., Wannamaker, L. and Quie, P.G. 1981. Potentiation of opsonization and phagocytosis of *Streptococcus pyogenes* following growth in the presence of clindamycin. J. Clin. Invest. 67: 1249-1256.

8   Gemmell, C.G., Peterson, P.K., Schmelling, D. and Quie, P.G. 1982. Studies on the potentiation of phagocytosis of *Streptococcus pyogenes* by treatment with various antibiotics. Drugs Exptl. Clin. Res. Vlll, 235-240.

9   Gemmell, C.G. Spear, T. and Peterson, P.K. 1983. Morphological changes in *Bacteroides fragilis* and *Klebsiella pneumoniae* attributable to growth in the presence of various antibiotics. Eur. J. Clin. Microbiol. 2: 217-221.

10 Hand, W.L., King-Thomson, N.L. and Johnson, J. 1984. Influence of bacterial-antibiotic interactions on subsequent antimicrobial activity of alveolar macrophages. J. Infect. Dis. 149: 271-276.

11 Howard, R.J. and Soucy, D.M. 1983. Potentiation of phagocytosis of *Bacteroides fragilis* following incubation with clindamycin. J. Antimicrob. Chemother. 12 (Suppl. C): 63-68.

12 Kasper, D.L. 1976. The polysaccharide capsule of
    Bacteroides fragilis subspecies *fragilis* :
    immunochemical and morphologic definition.
    J. Infect. Dis. 133: 79–87.

13 Kasper, D.L., Hayes, M.E., Reinap, B.G., Craft,
    F.O., Onderdonk, A.B. and Polk, B.F. 1977. Isolation
    and identification of encapsulated strains of
    Bacteroides fragilis. J. Infect. Dis. 136: 75–81.

14 Kasper, D.L., Onderdonk, A.B., Reinapp B.G. and
    Lindberg, A.A. 1980. Variations of *Bacteroides
    fragilis* with *in vitro* passage : presence of an outer
    membrane–associated glycan and loss of capsular
    antigen. J. Infect. Dis. 142: 750–756.

15 Klempner M.S. and Styrt, B. 1981. Clindamycin uptake
    by human neutrophils. J. Infect. Dis. 144: 472–479.

16 Onderdonk, A.B., Kasper, D.L., Cisneros, R.L. and
    Bartlett, J.G. 1977. The capsular polysaccharide of
    Bacteroides fragilis as a virulence factor:
    comparison of the pathogenic potential of encapsulated
    and unencapsulated strains. J. Infect. Dis. 136: 82–89.

17 Root, R.K., Isturiz, R., Molavi, A., Metcalf, J.A. and
    Malech, H.L. 1981. Interactions between antibiotics
    and human neutrophils in .the killing of staphylococci
    : studies with normal and cytochalasin B-treated
    cells. J. Clin. Invest. 67: 247–259.

18 Simon, G.L., Klempner, M.S., Kasper, D.L. and Gorbach,
    S.L. 1982. Alterations in opsonophagocytic killing by
    neutrophils of *Bacteroides fragilis* associated with
    animal and laboratory passage: effect of capsular
    polysaccharide. J. Infect. Dis. 145: 72–77.

19 Tofte, R.W., Peterson, P.K., Schmelling, D., Bracke,
    J., Kim, Y. and Quie, P.G. 1980. Opsonization of four
    Bacteroides species: role of the classical complement
    pathway and immunoglobulin. Infect. Immun. 27: 784–792.

20 Wade, B.H., Kasper, D.L. and Mandell, G.L. 1983.
    Interactions of *Bacteroides fragilis* and phagocytes:
    studies with whole organisms, purified capsular
    polysaccharide and clindamycin-treated bacteria.
    J. Antimicrob. Chemother. 12 (Suppl. C): 51–62.

CHAPTER 10

ANTIBIOTICS, ANAEROBES AND COLONIZATION RESISTANCE

D. van der Waaij

Laboratory for Medical Microbiology, University of Groningen, The Netherlands.

Contents

Introduction

Animal studies

References

INTRODUCTION

The introduction and widespread use of antibiotics has resulted in profound changes in the number and character of infections that are encountered. This was already evident in the sixties (22,15). Although the problem of staphylococcal infections still received considerable attention and emphasis from many workers in the early sixties, several groups of workers, including ourselves, became impressed by the increasing prevalence and seriousness of infections with Gram-negative bacilli (2). The great majority of these infections were seen in immuno-compromised patients (2,4). This led us to investigate this type of infections in an animal model, particularly with regard to prophylaxis of such infections.

ANIMAL STUDIES

Attempting to minimize infections in mice, immuno-logically compromised by whole body irradiation, we first attempted strict protective isolation, assuming that bacterial contamination from the environment and subsequent colonization of the intestinal tract might be the major cause of infection. The results were disappointing; neither the bacterial species isolated from the heart blood nor the mean survival time after irradiation differed between mice that had been isolated and control animals. This indicated that endogenous Gram-negative bacteria present at the time of admission into the isolator might be as virulent for irradiated mice as exogenous potentially pathogenic bacteria. Furthermore, the type of bacteria cultured from the heart blood at necropsy had the gastrointestinal tract as their normal habitat, which made it likely that the digestive tract was the major source of infection (1). Next, the effect of broad-spectrum systemic antibiotic administration for prophylaxis of infection was investigated. This approach resulted in some reduction of infections with Gram- negative species but this reduction was not significant.

As a third approach we tried to decontaminate the digestive tract before and for some time after irradiation to prevent infection. Oral administration of non-absorbable broad-spectrum antibiotics was found to be very effective. In successfully decontaminated mice, the median lethal irradiation dose and the mean survival time after irradiation increased, and were found to be identical to those in germ-free mice (3,7,9,18).

After this finding antibiotic decontamination was performed on a large scale in irradiation experiments. In the first months of large-scale application of antibiotic decontamination it was found that if decontaminated mice were accidentally contaminated with Gram-negative bacilli that were resistant to the antibiotics used for decontamination, such contamination usually spread extremely rapidly to all neighbouring cages containing decontaminated mice. This invariably caused the untimely death of animals in these cages that had been irradiated (21).

The results of these experiments and evidence from other work that oral treatment with broad-spectrum antibiotics might play a role in "overgrowth" with resistant bacteria led us to perform oral contamination experiments (11,19) in: (A) untreated mice with a conventional microflora; (B) mice that had been irradiated with a dose of low-lethality; and (C) mice that had been successfully decontaminated. Identical oral contamination doses had a completely different result in these three types of mice. In the untreated group of conventional animals, high oral doses were required for colonization to reach concentrations of $>10^3$ of the bacteria employed for experimental contamination per gram of faeces. Peak concentrations of $>10^5$ contaminants per gram of faeces were only seen for about two days following the highest contamination dose of 10^{11} contaminants. In the irradiated animals with a dose of low lethality, considerably higher average concentrations were seen, whereas in the decontaminated mice all contamination doses resulted in persistent, extremely high faecal concentrations ($>$ or $= 10^8$ bacteria per gram) of the contaminant. The difference between the first set of experiments and the third was the presence and the absence respectively of a resident microflora. Stepwise simplification of conventional flora by antibiotic treatment under isolation conditions indicated that the difference in response to oral contamination between experiment A and C was caused by the presence of anaerobic bacteria in mice in group A. This influence of the anaerobic part of the flora on the threshold dose for colonization with potentially pathogenic bacteria and the control of their numbers during colonization was called Colonization Resistance (CR) (14,19).

In mice irradiated with a dose of low-lethality the CR was also found to be somewhat decreased, but by far less than in the decontaminated animals. Microscopic investigation of the salivary glands and the intestinal mucosa indicated a marked reduction of activity of both the salivary glands and the goblet cells in the intestines.

Furthermore, the intestinal transit time was prolonged in the first week after irradiation, and the secretion of IgA into the intestinal lumen was significantly decreased for a period of almost 3 weeks (20).

In short, irradiation apparently interfered with the lubricating function of saliva and mucus and prolonged the transit of contents, and the reduced IgA secretion may have enhanced the adhesion of potentially pathogenic bacteria to the mucosa. Consequently, it was concluded that not only anaerobic bacteria but also host factors played a role in the CR of the digestive tract.

Because of the possible relevance of our findings in mice to clinical practice we subsequently investigated whether the bacteria that cause lethal infections in individuals with decreased resistance could be eliminated selectively from the alimentary tract microflora. Antimicrobial treatment should preferably result in complete suppression of all potentially pathogenic bacteria but leave the anaerobic microflora unaffected. For this purpose (selective decontamination, SD) drugs were selected which are known to affect anaerobes minimally or not at all. In the course of a series of screening experiments in mice it was found that, for oral application, nalidixic acid and other quinolones, co-trimoxazole, polymyxin, aztreonam, cephradine, nystatin and amphotericin B met this requirement (2,11,22). Tobramycin was found to be marginally applicable for SD because the dose that just suppressed the Gram-negative bacilli completely was only slightly lower than the dose at which the anaerobic micro-flora started to be effected obviously (8,18). These findings in mice appeared in subsequent studies to apply also in man (12,13).

In irradiation studies, selectively decontaminated mice appeared to survive longer after lethal irradiation and to have an LD_{50} for irradiation similar to that of successfully completely deconta- minated mice. This indicated that SD prevented infection without affecting the "natural threshold for contamination" constituted by the anaerobic flora associated part of CR. Later, propectively randomized studies in patients with acute leukemia showed that the findings in mice applied to man (1,10,21).

References

1   Dekker, A.W., Rozeberg-Arska, M., Sixma, J.J. and
     Verhoef, J. 1981 Prevention of infection by
     trimethoprim-sulfamethoxazole plus amphotericin B in
     patients with non-lymphocytic leukemia.
     Ann. Int. Med. 95: 555-559.

2   Emmelot, C.H. and Van der Waaij, D. 1980 The dose
     at which neomycin and polymyxin B can be applied for
     selective decontamination of the digestive tract in
     mice. J. Hyg. 84: 331-340.

3   Finland, M. 1970 Changing ecology of bacterial
     infections as related to antibacterial therapy.
     J. Inf. Dis. 122: 419-431.

4   Frei,E., Levin,R.H., Bodey, G.P., Morse, E.E. and
     Freireich, E.J. 1965 The nature and control of
     infections in patients with acute leukemia.
     Cancer Research 25: 1511-1515.

5   McCabe, W.R. and Jackson, G.G. 1962 Gram-negative
     bacteremia. I. Etiology and ecology.
     Arch. Intern. Med. 110: 847-855.

6   McLaughlin,M.M. Dacquisto,M.P., Jacobus, D.P. and
     Horowitz, R.E. 1964 Effects of the germfree state
     on response of mice to wholebody irradiation.
     Radiat. Res. 23: 333-349.

7   McLaughlin, M.M., Woodward, K.T. and Stromberg, L.R.
     1971 Effects of the germfree state on the response of
     mice exposed to neutrongamma radiation.
     Radiat. Res. 35: 559-560.

8   Mulder, J.G., Wiersma, W.E., Welling, G.W. and Van der
     Waaij, D. 1984 Low dose oral tobramycin treatment for
     selective decontamination of the digestive tract: a
     study in human volunteers.
     J. Antimicrob. Chemother. 13: 495-504.

9   Myerowitz, R.L., Medeiros, A.A. and O'Brien, T.F.
     1971 Recent experience with bacillemia due to Gram-
     negative organisms. J. Inf. Dis. 124: 239-246.

10   Sleijfer, D.T., Mulder, N.H., De Vries-Hospers, H.G.,
     Fidler, V., Nieweg, H.O., Van der Waaij, D. and Van
     Saene, H.K.F. 1980 Infection prevention in
     granulocytopenic patients by selective decontamination
     of the digestive tract. Eur. J. Cancer 16: 859-869.

11   Thijm, H.A. and Van der Waaij, D. 1979 The effect of
     three frequently applied antibiotics on the
     colonization resistance of the digestive tract of
     mice. J. Hyg. 82: 397-405.

12   De Vries-Hospers, H.G., Welling, G.W., Swabb, E.A. and
     Van der Waaij, D. 1984 Selective decontamination of
     the digestive tract with aztreonam: a study of 10
     healthy volunteers. J. Inf. Dis. 10: 636-642.

13   De Vries-Hospers, H.G., Welling, G.W. and·Van der
     Waaij, D.   1985   Norfloxacin for selective
     decontamination: a study in human volunteers. In:
     B.S. Wostmann (ed.) Germfree Research: microflora
     control and its application to the biomedical
     sciences.   Allan R. Liss Inc. New York, p. 259-262.

14   Van der Waaij, D., Berghuis-de Vries, J.M. and
     Lekkerkerk- Van der Wees, J.E.C.   1971   Colonization
     resistance of the digestive tract in conventional and
     antibiotic-treated mice. J. Hyg.   69: 405-411.

15   Van der Waaij, D. and Berghuis, J.M.   1974
     Determination of the colonization resistance of the
     digestive tract of individual mice.
     J. Hyg. 72: 379-387.

16   Van der Waaij, D. and Heidt, P.J.   1977   Intestinal
     bacterial ecology in relation to immunological factors
     and   other defense mechanisms. In: L. Hambraens, L.A.
     Hanson and H. McFarlane (eds.).   Food and Immunology.
     Almqvist and Wiksell International Stockholm. p. 133-141.

17   Van der Waaij, D., Tielemans-Speltie, T.M. and De
     Rouck-Houben, A.M.J.   1978   Relation between the
     faecal concentration of various potentially pathogenic
     microorganisms and infections in individuals (mice)
     with   severely decreased resistance to infection.
     Antonie v. Leeuwenhoek .44: 395-405.

18   Van der Waaij D. Aberson J., Thijm, A.H. and Welling
     G.W.   1982 The screening of four aminoglycosides in
     the   selective decontamination of the digestive tract
     in mice.   Infection   10: 35-40.

19   Van der Waaij, D. and Van der Waaij, J.M.   1985
     Spread of multiresistant Gram-negative bacilli among
     severely immuno- compromised mice during prophylactic
     treatment with different oral antimicrobial drugs.
     In: B.S. Wostmann (ed.) Germfree Research:
     microflora control and its application to the
     biomedical sciences,   Allen, R. Liss.Inc. New York
     p.245-250.

20   Walburg, H.E., Myatt, E.J. and Robie, D.M.   1968   The
     effect of strain and diet on the thirty-day mortality
     of X-irradiated germfree mice.
     Radiat. Res.   27: 616-629.

21   Wade, J.C., De Jongh, C.A., Newman, K.A., Crowley, J.,
     Wiernik, P.H. and Schimpff, S.C.   1983   Selective
     antimicrobial modulation as prophylaxis against
     infection during granulocytopenia: trimethoprim-
     sulfamethoxazole versus nalidixic acid.
     J. Inf. Dis. 147: 624-634.

22   Wiegersma, N.,Jansen, G. and Van der Waaij, D.   1982
     The effect of twelve antimicrobial drugs on the
     colonization resistance of the digestive tract of
     mice.   Journal of Hygiene 88: 221-230.

23   Wilson, B.R.   1963   Survival studies of whole body X-
     irradiated germfree (axenic) mice. Radiat. Res. 20:   477-483.

CHAPTER 11

ANTIBIOTIC MANIPULATION OF THE RUMEN MICROFLORA.   THE EFFECTS OF

AVOPARCIN AND MONENSIN ON THE RELEASE OF TRITIUM FROM LABELLED

CELLULOSE BY *BACTEROIDES SUCCINOGENES* AND THE RUMEN FUNGUS

NEOCALLIMASTIX FRONTALIS.

C.S. Stewart, Sylvia H. Duncan and *K.N. Joblin

Rowett Research Institute, Bucksburn, Aberdeen, AB2 9SB, U.K.
and *DSIR, Palmerston North, New Zealand.

Contents

Abstract

Introduction

Materials and methods

    Cultures and media

    Tritiation, radioactive counting
    and chemical determinations

    Antibiotics

    Inoculum preparation

        a) adaptation

        b) counts

Results

    Adaptation of *Bacteroides succinogenes*

    The effects of avoparcin and monensin
    on cellulolysis by *B. succinogenes*

    Adaptation of *Neocallimastix frontalis*

    The effect of avoparcin and monensin
    on cellulolysis by *N. frontalis*

Discussion

References

ABSTRACT

Studies were made on the effects of avoparcin and monensin on the rate of release of radioactivity from reductively tritiated cellulose by *Bacteroides succinogenes* and *Neocallimastix frontalis*. Monensin reduced the activity of *B. succinogenes* and *N. frontalis* markedly when present at >8 mcg/ml (*B. succinogenes*) or > 2mcg/ml (*N.frontalis*). Avoparcin was only marginally inhibitory to *B.succinogenes* when present at < 32mcg/ml, and appeared to slightly enhance the attack of labelled cellulose by *N. frontalis*.

INTRODUCTION

The changes in the rumen fermentation that accompany the addition of monensin or avoparcin to the diet of ruminants are thought to stem largely from decreased methanogenesis, a consequence of the supression of growth of a number of Gram-positive bacteria (and possibly some protozoa) that possess hydrogenases and thereby normally supply hydrogen for methanogenesis by interspecies transfer (20). When methanogenesis is reduced, propionate serves as an electron sink, and the combination of reduced methanogenesis and increased propionate production results in improved retention of carbon and energy in the rumen fermentation (19). The evidence for this scenario is based mainly on experiments with axenic cultures *in vitro* (4,6,7,12), incubation of mixed rumen contents *in vitro* (18,19), and experiments *in vivo* (reviewed by Chalupa, 3).

Enhanced propionate production could benefit animals fed low quality roughages, which typically support acetogenic fermentations (5). Although it is known that antibiotics affect rumen functions such as proteolysis and deamination, their effects on plant cell wall digestion are not entirely clear (3). Most studies *in vitro* have concentrated on factors affecting the extent rather than rate of cellulolysis (7,13). For example, when cellulose degradation by *B. succinogenes* was tested after incubation for 7 days, it was found that significant digestion occurred in the presence of avoparcin at concentrations up to 64 mcg/ml(13); such long incubations could however mask more dramatic effects of antibiotics on the rate of cellulolysis. Although rumen phycomycete fungi such as *Neocallimastix frontalis* are assumed to have an important role in plant cell wall digestion in the rumen (9), their responses to animal feed antibiotics have not previously been reported.

Tritiated cellulose has been successfully used in the detection and enumeration of cellulolytic anaerobes (14,16). This paper describes the use of tritiated cellulose in a rapid comparative study of the effects of avoparcin and monensin on the rate of degradation of cellulose by *B.succinogenes*, the predominant cellulolytic bacterium of ruminants fed monensin and avoparcin (1,13), and by the rumen fungus *N. frontalis*. Since it is known that rumen micro-organisms increase their tolerance of antibiotics by adaptation (4,12), the experiments were performed with cultures adapted to growth in the presence of the relevant antibiotics.

MATERIAL AND METHODS

<u>Cultures and media</u>.　*B. succinogenes* strain BL2 and

N. frontalis strain PNK2 were isolated as previously described (15,8). Media were prepared and maintained by the anaerobic procedure of Bryant (2), using 16 x 150mm culture tubes containing 10ml of medium and sealed with butyl rubber septum stoppers (Bellco Glass Inc., New Jersey, U.S.A.). *B. succinogenes* was maintained on the HSM medium of Stewart *et al* (15), with cellobiose 0.25% w/v as substrate. *N. frontalis* was maintained on HSM medium, containing D-glucose 0.2% w/v and agar 0.1% w/v. The initial pH of the media was from 6.7-6.9. When required, labelled cellulose (below) replaced sugars and agar and was added to the medium at a final concentration of 1mg/ml. Incubations were at $39° + 1°C$.

Tritiation, radioactive counting and chemical determinations. Methods used for reductive tritiation of phosphoric acid-swollen cellulose (Avicel pH 105, Honeywell & Stein, Wallington, UK), for radioactive counting and for the determination of the specific activity of cellulose were those previously used (13).

Antibiotics. Avoparcin sulphate was from Cyanamid (GB) Ltd, Gosport, Hants, U.K. Sodium monensin was from The Lilly Research Centre Ltd, Windlesham, Surrey, U.K. Filter-sterilised concentrated stock solutions of the antibiotics, prepared as previously described (7,12) were added to autoclaved media (121°C, 15 min) immediately before inoculation with the organism under study.

Inoculum preparation.

a) Adaptation. *B. succinogenes* strain BL2 was adapted to monensin or avoparcin by cultivation in HSM medium containing cellobiose (above) and the highest concentration of antibiotic (16 mcg/ml avoparcin or 1 mcg/ml monensin) that could be tolerated by previously unexposed cultures

(7,12). Inocula were grown for 16-18 h and had an optical density (measured spectrophotometrically at 540 nm) of >0.7, with at least 1 x 10⁸ viable cells/ml. *N. frontalis* was adapted in HSM medium with agar and glucose (above), and either avoparcin (8 mcg/ml) or monensin (1 mcg/ml). Inocula were grown for 72 h and contained at least 1 x 10⁴ zoospores/ml.

b) <u>Counts</u>. The numbers of viable bacteria or fungal zoospores in inocula were determined by the rapid radiometric method of Stewart *et al.* (14).

RESULTS

<u>Adaptation of *B. succinogenes*</u>. When *B.succinogenes* strain BL2 which had not previously been exposed to antibiotics

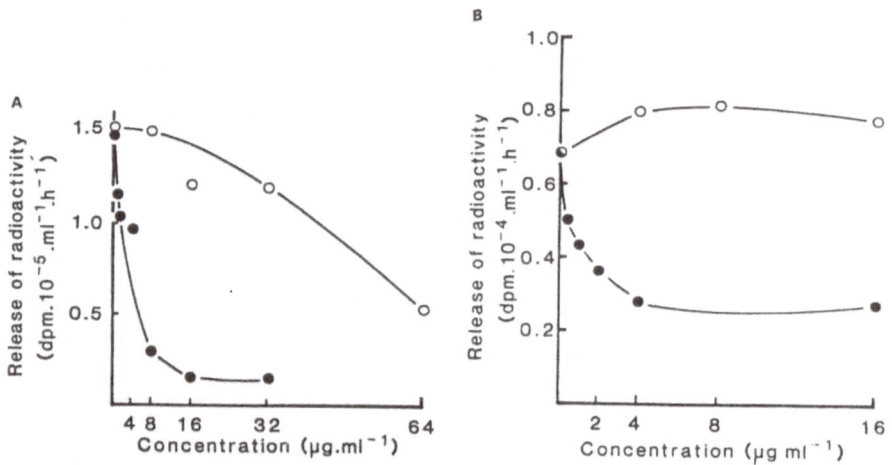

Fig. 1. The effect of avoparcin and monensin on the maximum rate of release of radioactivity from tritiated cellulose by adapted cultures of a) *B. succinogenes* strain BL2, and b) *N. frontalis* strain PNK2. Broths containing tritiated cellulose and antibiotics at the concentrations indicated were inoculated with adapted cultures, and the maximum rate of release of radioactivity was determined between 4 and 5h (*B. succinogenes*) or 24 and 48h (*N. frontalis*) after inoculation, see Materials and methods. ● = monensin; O = avoparcin. Each point is the average of three separate determinations.

was grown in cellobiose broths containing avoparcin or monensin, good growth (540 OD >0.7) was obtained in the presence of avoparcin at 16 mcg/ml or monensin at 1 mcg/ml. On first exposure, monensin caused an extended lag period, but serial transfers on to fresh media containing the drug abolished this effect, as in an earlier study (7). However, growth in the presence of monensin at a concentration of 2 mcg/ml or more was relatively weak (540 OD from 0.5 - 0.6) and so cultures grown in the presence of 1 mcg/ml monensin (540 OD 0.75) were used to inoculate the broths containing tritiated cellulose.

Avoparcin at 16 mcg/ml had little effect on growth once the cultures had been exposed to the drug (12), so this concentration was used for the preparation of inocula. The effects of avoparcin and monensin on cellulolysis by B. succinogenes. Incubation of *B. succinogenes* strain BL2 with tritiated cellulose resulted in the release of radio-activity into the culture supernates as previously described for *B. succinogenes* strain Bac 20 (13). Measure-ment of the activity released at hourly intervals for up to 10h showed that the maximum rate of release of activity occurred between 4 and 5h after inoculation. The increase in radioactive counts in the culture supernates during this period was therefore used to compare the effects of avoparcin and monensin on the degradation of cellulose. The results of these tests, summarised in Fig. 1a, showed that monensin was much more inhibitory than avoparcin to the release of radioactivity from labelled cellulose by *B. succinogenes*.

To test whether the release of radioactivity correlated with cellulose solubilisation, the specific radioactivity of residual cellulose in cultures without the antibiotics was measured at intervals during a 6h incubation period. At 2, 3, 4, 5 and 6h after inoculation with strain BL2, the specific activity of cellulose residues was 97, 96, 89, 88 and 90% respectively of the initial value (0.9 x 10^6 dpm/mg). The maximum rate of release of radioactivity by *B. succinogenes* corresponded to a rate of cellulose solubilisation of around 1-5 mg/h.

<u>Adaptation of *N. frontalis*</u>. When *N. frontalis* strain PNK2 was grown on glucose, avoparcin (8 mcg/ml) had no detectable effect on growth (measured as the number of viable zoospores/ml after incubation for 72 h). At a concentration of 2 mcg/ml, monensin reduced the numbers of zoospores present, so the inocula were prepared in media containing either avoparcin at 8 mcg/ml, or monensin at 1 mcg/ml.

<u>The effects of avoparcin and monensin on cellulolysis by *N. frontalis*</u>. When *N. frontalis* was incubated with labelled cellulose, measurement of the radioactivity released at intervals of 8 - 12h during 72h incubations showed that the maximum rate of release was attained between 24 and 48h after inoculation with the fungus. The change in radioactive counts in the culture supernates between 24 and 48h after inoculation with *N. frontalis* was therefore used to calculate the rate of release of radio-activity.

The effects of monensin and avoparcin on the maximum rate of release of radioactivity from labelled cellulose by *N. frontalis* strain PNK2 are summarised in Fig. 1b. Avoparcin appeared to have a slightly stimulatory effect, whereas monensin was clearly inhibitory. The specific activity of the residual cellulose in cultures without the antibiotics was 0.6 x 10^6 dpm/mg immediately after inoculation with the fungus, and 0.7×10^6 dpm/mg after incubation for 48h. The rate of release of radioactivity in cultures without antibiotics corresponded to a rate of cellulose solubilisation of around 0.1mg/h a much slower rate than that calculated for *B. succinogenes* (above).

DISCUSSION

When amorphous cellulose is reduced with tritiated KBH (4) under alkaline conditions, the terminal glucose units at the reducing ends of the cellulose molecules are converted to the alcohol glucitol, bearing tritiated primary alcohol groups (10, 16). The action of cellulases releases glucitol into the medium, possibly attached to short chain oligosaccharides (16). From the present study it appears that the ends of the cellulose chains were preferentially solubilised by *B. succinogenes*, because the specific activity of the cellulose dropped during incubation with this organism. Previous studies have found no evidence for extensive exchange of tritium between labelled cellulose and the medium at the pH values employed here (16). Preferential solubilisation may be a consequence of the accessibility of the ends of the cellulose chains to the bacterium, however it may also reflect the mode of attack of labelled cellulose by the cellulases of *B.succinogenes*. The cellulases of *N. frontalis* may act differently, in that the specific activity of the cellulose residues appeared to be marginally increased during attack. Experiments with purified cellulases would be needed to clarify this point.

The effects of avoparcin and monensin on the rate of release of tritium by *B. succinogenes* were broadly consistent with previous findings on the effect of avoparcin on the extent of cellulose solubilisation (13) and the effect of avoparcin (12) and monensin (4) on growth. It is possible, however, that in the natural environment further adaptive resistance could be developed over a long period of exposure; by analogy with processes known to occur in other habitats (11) the aquisition of resistance by horizontal gene flow from other rumen species might also occur.

The anaerobic fungus *N. frontalis* was much less active in releasing radioactivity from labelled cellulose than was *B. succinogenes*. It seemed that the invasive growth form of the fungus (9) may be better suited to the colonisation of large pieces of plant material, in contrast to the small particles (20 nm) used here. *N. frontalis* was more sensitive to monensin than was *B. succinogenes*, but the results of these experiments suggest that such fungi may play a predominant role in cellulolysis in the rumen of animals fed avoparcin.

In ruminants fed antibiotics, the concentration of antibiotics in the rumen would probably be at the lower end of the ranges studied here. Factors affecting the concentration of additives *in vivo* include the amount present in the diet, solubility in water, the rumen volume and the turnover rate of the rumen contents. Wallace *et al* (19) calculated that in sheep of rumen volume 4 litres, turnover rate 1.2/d, fed 1.2 kg/d of a diet containing monensin at 10 mg/kg, the average concentration of monensin in the rumen contents would be *ca* 2.5 mcg/ml. Avoparcin is normally added to the diet at *ca* 33 mg/kg so under similar conditions, the average concentration of avoparcin in the rumen would be *ca* 8 mcg/ml.

Finally, as some antibiotics extend the residence

time of the dietary solids in the ruminant gut (3), they allow more time for digestion to occur. It is known that the rumen fungi reduce the particle size of plant material (9), and that the residence time of plant material in the gut is inversely related to particle size, with only the smallest particles passing out of the rumen (17). The reduction by monensin of plant cell wall breakdown by rumen fungi, described in this study, could contribute to the enhanced residence time of plant material in the gut of ruminants fed this antibiotic. How important and widespread such effects are remains to be evaluated.

ACKNOWLEDGEMENT

We thank Cyanamid (GB) for a grant in aid of this research.

References

1   Brulla, W.J. and Bryant, M.P. 1980 Monensin-induced
     changes in the major species of the rumen bacterial
     population. Abstr. 80th Ann. Meeting ASM, 1121.

2   Bryant, M.P. 1972 Commentary on the Hungate
     technique for culture of anaerobic bacteria.
     Am. J. Clin. Nutr. 25: 1324-1328.

3   Chalupa, W. 1984 Manipulation of rumen
     fermentation. In: W. Haresign and D.J.A. Cole (eds.),
     Recent advances in animal nutrition, Butterworths,
     London. pp.143-160.

4   Chen, J. and Wolin, M.J. 1979 Effect of monensin
     and lasalocid-sodium on the growth of methanogenic and
     rumen saccharolytic bacteria.
     Appl. Environ. Microbiol. 38: 72-77.

5   Church, D.C. 1984 Livestock feeds and feeding. O
     and B Books   Corvallis.

6   Dennis, S.M., Nagaraja, T.G. and Bartley, E.E. 1981
     Effects of lasalocid or monensin on lactate producing
     or using rumen bacteria. J. Anim. Sci. 52: 418-426.

7   Henderson, C., Stewart, C.S. and Nekrep, F.V. 1981
     The effect of monensin on pure and mixed cultures of
     rumen bacteria. J. Appl. Bacteriol. 51: 159-169.

8   Joblin, K.N. 1981 Isolation, enumeration and
     maintenance of rumen anaerobic fungi in roll tubes.
     Appl. Environ. Microbiol. 41: 1119-1122.

9   Orpin, C. G. 1984 The role of ciliate protozoa and
     fungi in the rumen digestion of plant cell walls.
     Anim. Fd Sci. Technol. 10: 121-143.

10   Paart, E. and Samuelson, O. 1970 Determination and
     identification of aldehyde end groups in cellulose.
     Carb. Res. 15: 111-121.

11   Sherratt, D.J. 1982 The maintenance and propagation
     of plasmid genes in bacterial populations.
     J. Gen. Microbiol. 128: 655-661.

12   Stewart, C.S., Crossley, M.V. and Garrow, S.H. 1983
     The effect of avoparcin on laboratory cultures of
     rumen bacteria.
     Eur. J. Appl. Microbiol. Biotechnol. 17: 292-297.

13   Stewart, C.S. and Duncan, S.H. 1985 The effect of
     avoparcin on cellulolytic bacteria of the ovine rumen.
     J. Gen. Microbiol. 131: 427-435.

14   Stewart, C.S., Duncan, S.H. and Joblin, K.N. 1985
     The use of tritiated cellulose for the rapid
     enumeration of cellulolytic anaerobes. Lett. Appl.
     Microbiol. (In press.)

15   Stewart, C.S., Paniagua, C., Dinsdale, D., Cheng, K-J.
     and Garrow, S.H. 1981   Selective isolation and
     characteristics of *Bacteroides succinogenes* from the
     rumen of a cow. Appl. Environ. Microbiol. 41: 504-510.

16   Stewart, J.C. Stewart, C.S. and Heptinstall, J.   1982
     The use of tritiated cellulose in screening for
     cellulolytic microorganisms.
     Biotechnol. Lett. 4: 459-464.

17   Ullyat, M.J., Dellow, D.W., John, A., Reid, C.S.W. and
     Waghorn, G.C. 1985   The contribution of chewing,
     during eating   and rumination, to the clearance of
     digesta from the reticulo-rumen. In: L.P. Milligan and
     W.L. Grovum (ed.). Proc. 6th Int. Symp. on Ruminant
     Physiology. (In the press).

18   Van Nevel, C.J. and Demeyer, D.I.   1977   Effect of
     monensin on rumen metabolism *in vitro*.
     Appl. Environ. Microbiol 34: 251-257.

19   Wallace, R.J., Czerkawski, J.W. and Breckenridge, G.
     1981 Effect of monensin on the fermentation of basal
     rations in the rumen simulation technique (Rusitec).
     Br. J. Nutr. 46: 131-148.

20   Wolin, M.J. 1982   Hydrogen transfer in microbial
     communities. In: A.T.Bull and J.H. Slater (eds.),
     Interactions and communities. Academic Press. London.
     pp.323-356.

SECTION 4. ADVANCES IN GENETIC MANIPULATION AND THE COMMERCIAL EXPLOITATION OF ANAEROBES.

Co-Chairman of Session : Dr. D.B. Archer and J.M.Hardie.

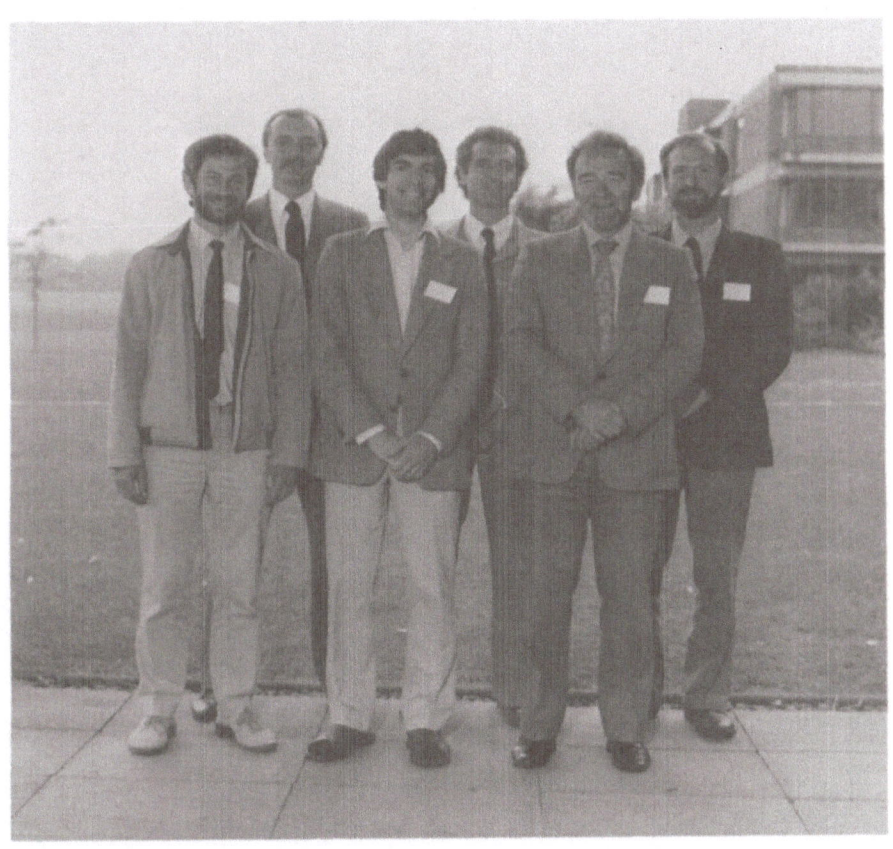

From left to right :

D.B. Archer, R. Sleat, N.F. Fairweather, G.P. Hazlewood,
W.A. Hamilton and J.M. Hardie.

CHAPTER 12

GENETIC APPROACHES WITH METHANOGENS IMPORTANT IN MESOPHILIC ANAEROBIC DIGESTION

Jane E. Harris, D. M. Evans, Margaret R. Knox and D. B. Archer

AFRC Food Research Institute-Norwich, Colney Lane, Norwich NR4 7UA

Contents

Abstract

Introduction.

Role of methanogens in anaerobic digestion.

    Microbiology of anaerobic digestion

    Methanogenic species occurring in mesophilic anaerobic digesters

Genetic manipulation of methanogens important in mesophilic anaerobic digestion.

    Potential for genetic manipulation of methanogens

    Genetic status of methanogens

    Initial aims and problems

Progress.

    Isolation of genetically marked strains

    Protoplast formation

    Vectors

Prospects and conclusions.

References

ABSTRACT

The methanogens are strictly anaerobic archaebacteria which utilize hydrogen or acetate for the production of methane. They are of biotechnological importance since their activities are rate-limiting in the anaerobic digestion of soluble wastes; removal of hydrogen controls the degradation of volatile fatty acids such as propionic and butyric while removal of acetate controls the pH within the digester. The anaerobic digestion process may be improved by genetic manipulation of the methanogens and thus our work is directed towards developing gene-transfer systems in both hydrogenotrophic (*Methanobacterium, Methanobrevibacter*) and acetotrophic (*Methanosarcina*) species occurring in mesophilic anaerobic digesters.

Initial aims are to

a) isolate genetically marked strains,

b) produce protoplasts for DNA extraction, transformation and fusion,

c) isolate plasmids and phages of methanogens as potential cloning vectors.

INTRODUCTION

The attractions of treating commercial wastes by anaerobic digestion are obvious; effluent charges are markedly reduced and methane is produced which is a valuable by-product. The process is potentially cost effective, and particularly so if high treatment rates can be achieved but this, in turn, can lead to unreliability. One approach to optimizing anaerobic digestion is through improved process control and digester design, but ultimately the process depends on the co-ordinated activities of the inter-dependent microbial species involved. We must look, therefore, to a better understanding of the microbiology of anaerobic digestion as a means of increasing efficiency and reliability, and this raises the prospect of using genetically 'tailored' strains of methanogens.

ROLE OF METHANOGENS IN ANAEROBIC DIGESTION

Microbiology of anaerobic digestion. The degradation of complex organic matter to methane requires a complex mixture of bacterial species (11). In the degradation of soluble organic matter it is the terminal, methanogenic reactions which are the slowest steps (1,13). Approximately 70% of the methane produced is from acetic acid, the remainder being derived from the reduction of carbon dioxide by hydrogen : removal of acetic acid by the methanogenic bacteria regulates pH within a digester and removal of hydrogen facilitates the degradation of higher volatile fatty acids (1,13). The most common cause of failure in anaerobic digesters is acidification, accompanied by an increase in hydrogen levels, so it is the methanogenic bacteria, both acetate-utilizing and hydrogen-utilizing, which deserve detailed attention.

Methanogenic species occurring in mesophilic anaerobic digesters. The methanogens are a physiologically diverse group whose members inhabit niches encompassing a wide variety of physical and chemical conditions (3). Species commonly found as the predominant methanogens in mesophilic anaerobic digesters are from the genera *Methanobacterium, Methanobrevibacter, Methanospirillum* (all hydrogen-utilizers), *Methanosarcina* and *Methanothrix* (both acetate-utilizers). Anaerobic techniques allow the isolation and cultivation of pure cultures of most species observed in anaerobic digesters, although the acetate-utilizing *Methanothrix* can prove refractory.

GENETIC MANIPULATION OF METHANOGENS IMPORTANT IN MESOPHILIC ANAEROBIC DIGESTION

Potential for genetic manipulation of methanogens. As the rate-limiting organisms in anaerobic digesters, the methanogens are an obvious microbiological target for optimizing the process. Improvements in treatment rates and reliability should be achieved by maintaining increased methanogenic activity in the digester and various means of attaining this objective are suggested in Table 1. Genetic techniques have the potential to fulfil some of these criteria.

Table 1. Targets for producing improved strains of methanogens by genetic breeding

Aims	Desirable properties of improved strains
1. Increase methanogen biomass in the digester.	Adhesion, aggregation and flocculation.
2. Increase activity per unit weight of methanogen biomass	Overproduction of appropriate enzymes, e.g. regulatory mutants. Increased affinity of enzyme for substrate.
3. Extend substrate range for methanogenesis	Methane from propionate and butyrate.
4. Produce strains of methanogen tolerant to perturbation of digester conditions.	Tolerance to extremes of pH and toxic compounds, e.g. heavy metals, ammonia,

Genetic status of methanogens. Historically, genetic studies with methanogens are very recent, beginning in 1982 (8,28). Most research has been with those species which are more amenable to culture and genetic techniques, such as *Methanobacterium thermoautotrophicum* and the marine methanococci. Relatively little research has been carried out with the mesophilic methanogens found in digesters.

All reports of genome size in methanogens indicate that these are comparable to those of typical prokaryotes (21,27) and the range of DNA base ratios (27 to 61 moles %G+C) illustrates the diversity of the group. In the absence of endogenous cloning systems, methanogen genes have been isolated from genomic libraries prepared in *Escherichia coli*, and include genes for ribosomal and transfer RNAs (17,18,32), for subunits of the DNA-dependent RNA polymerase (9) and methyl coenzyme M reductase enzymes (22), and several which were selected by their ability to complement known auxotrophic mutations in *E. coli* (14,33). Sequencing of functionally expressed DNA fragments from the mesophilic marine species *Methanococcus voltae* (9) and *Methanococcus vannielii* (32), and from *Methanobrevibacter smithii* (15), has shown that non-repetitive A-T rich regions occur between genes, possibly functioning as gene spacers, but it is not yet known if this is a genetic feature common to all methanogens. Although methanogen DNA is expressed efficiently in *E. coli*, it is unlikely that methanogen transcription signals are recognised by the eubacterial transcription apparatus, since the structure of all archaebacterial DNA-dependent RNA polymerases is distinct from the eubacterial enzymes (34). Methanogen promoter sequences are yet to be defined, but it is conceivable that transcription of methanogen DNA in *E.coli* occurs fortuitously by recognition of the A-T rich regions as eubacterial- like promoters (15). On the other hand, there is strong evidence for homologous translation signals since methanogens possess similar mRNA binding sites to eubacteria (9,15), and this would promote efficient hetero-logous expression. Examination of the structure of polyadenylated mRNA of *Methanococcus vannielii* has shown that it resembles eubacterial rather than eukaryotic mRNAs (10), and physical mapping has also indicated that methanogens employ the eubacterial operon system of gene organization (15,22,32). Despite these eubacterial features, it is possible that introns, a eukaryotic characteristic, may be found in methanogens in view of the fact that they occur in tRNAs of thermoacidophilic archaebacteria (19).

Mutants of *Methanobacterium thermoautotrophicum* and *Methanococcus voltae* have been induced by gamma radiation (7) and nitrosoguanidine (20) respectively, but optimum conditions for mutagenesis were not determined. To date, conjugation and transduction have not been demonstrated, although cryptic plasmids (25,31) and phages of methanogens are now known (5); however, calcium-induced transformation of *Methanococcus voltae* by linear chromosomal DNA has been observed (G. Bertani; personal communication). Meile *et al* (26) have prepared a series of recombinant plasmids derived from pME2001 of *Methanobacterium thermoautotrophicum* which are potential shuttle vectors for methanogens, but a major barrier to plasmid-mediated transformation in methanobacterial species is the absence of protoplast formation and regeneration. There are no reports of genetic instability in methanogens, although physical mapping and sequence studies have identified an insertion element in *Methanobrevibacter smithii* (15). An important consideration for the development of gene transfer is the occurrence of DNA restriction and modification systems. So far, restriction enzymes have only been detected in *Methanococcus aeolicus* (30), but other methanogens have not been systematically examined.

It would appear from the current information that gene structure and expression in methanogens follows eubacterial precedents, but methods for gene transfer in methanogens are badly needed to facilitate genetic studies in an archaebacterial cell environment.

Initial aims and problems.   Recombinant DNA technology undoubtedly offers the greatest scope for genetic 'tailoring' of industrially important micro-organisms.   As a pre-requisite for developing gene transfer in both hydrogenotrophic and acetotrophic methanogens important in anaerobic digestion, our initial aims are to isolate genetically-marked strains, generate protoplasts and develop cloning vectors.   The species relevant to our studies, however, possess a number of characteristics which present considerable difficulties for the geneticist. These are summarized in Table 2.   Physiological barriers

Table 2. Characteristics of methanogens that affect genetic studies

Characteristics	Consequence to genetics
1. Physiological.	
a) Obligate anaerobes	Require Eh – 300 mV
b) Long doubling times	Colony formation in 1–4 weeks
c) Poorly characterized	Lack of information
2. Morphological.	
a) Filamentous	No genetically
b) Aggregating	pure units
3. Archaebacterial.	
a) Insensitivity to inhibitors of cell wall and protein synthesis and RNA polymerase	Lack of resistance markers No enrichment for auxotrophs No L-forms
b) Novel cell walls insensitive to enzymic degradation	No lysis for DNA extraction No protoplast formation

are being overcome by the availability of improved anaerobic techniques, a better knowledge of the organisms and choice of the fastest growing strains, but the time scale of experiments will always be prolonged. The filamentous or aggregating morphology of the organisms will delay the segregation of genetically pure, mutant clones and this may be complicated further if methanogens are multi-genomic. Continued selective pressure should achieve segregation of dominant and recessive resistance markers, but for the isolation of auxotrophic mutants, the expression time allowed following mutagenesis will be critical, and effective enrichment methods valuable.

The archaebacterial characteristics and unique properties of methanogens are well documented (3,4), and the problems they pose to genetic studies are major ones. A variety of inhibitors with methanogen-specific target sites are needed for the isolation of useful resistant mutants, and those effective against cell-wall biosynthesis would be an especially valuable tool. Enzymes which degrade the pseudomurein and heteropolysaccharide cell wall types unique to methanogens are not yet available for protoplast formation and DNA extraction. Recently, however, autolytic activity has been demonstrated in culture supernatants of *Methanobacterium wolfei* (23) and *Methanosarcina mazei* (24) and these strains may provide a source of such enzymes.

PROGRESS

Isolation of genetically marked strains. Our studies have focussed on strains of hydrogenotrophic *Methanobacterium* and *Methanobrevibacter* species and the acetotrophic species *Methanosarcina mazei*, which show relatively short doubling times and acceptable plating efficiencies on solid medium.

As a prelude to the selection of resistant mutants, we determined the spectrum of *in vivo* antibiotic-sensitivity of methanogens. The activity of the most effective anti-biotics is shown in table 3, and illustrates the limited number of useful inhibitors available. It should also be

Table 3. Antibiotics and analogues of DNA bases and nucleosides inhibitory to methanogens in disc diffusion test.

| | Diameter of zone of inhibition (mms) at 1 mg/ml | | | |
	1	2	3	4
Bacitracin	35	38	63	−
Anisomycin	40	37	34	−
Gentamicin	37	41	−	−
Neomycin	−	−	−	22
Puromycin	16	18	16	23
Chloramphenicol	27	30	25	31
Lasalocid	25	30	22	28
Gramicidin	27	32	29	17
Metronidazole	22	25	21	18
6−mercaptopurine	45	60	15*	−
8−azaguanine	23	25	−	−
5−fluorouracil	48	12	11	−
7−deazaadenosine	23	35	−	−

1. *Methanobacterium* sp. strain FR-2, 2. *Methanobacterium bryantii*,
3. *Methanobrevibacter smithii*, 4. *Methanosarcina mazei*
* Diameter of zone at 10 mg/ml
− No zone

pointed out that the mode of action of antibiotics against methanogens is not always known and cannot be assumed to be identical to that in eubacteria; for example, chloramphenicol is unable to inhibit protein synthesis in methanogens (29) but exerts its effect through the oxidizing activity of an aryl nitro group (6). These factors should be considered when attempting to isolate resistant mutants. In an attempt to broaden the range of useful inhibitors we have tested analogues of amino acids and vitamins and found them to be ineffective at practicable concentrations, but some analogues of DNA bases and nucleosides are inhibitory (Table 3). Spontaneous mutants resistant to bacitracin (16), anisomycin, 6-mercaptopurine, 5-fluorouracil and 8-azaguanine have been selected and are being characterized to assess their suitability as genetic markers. Multiply-marked strains have also been isolated.

The strategy for developing genetic engineering in any micro- organism requires an efficient means of generating mutants. In agreement with Kiener *et al* (20) our investigations with *Methanobacterium* sp. strain FR-2 have shown that the lethal effect of nitrosoguanidine is enhanced by reducing agents in the medium. Work is in progress to compare mutation frequencies in the presence and absence of reducing agents, different buffer systems and at varying pH.

Protoplast formation. Extensive screening of commercially available carbohydrases and proteases, as well as bacteria and fungi from culture collections and isolated from sewage-treated soil, has failed to demonstrate lytic activity which might be used to produce protoplasts of methanogens. Surprisingly, the most significant progress has been made with the aggregate-forming *Methanosarcinaceae* which possess hetero-polysaccharide cell walls up to 200nm thick. A gas vacuolate strain of *Methanosarcina barkeri* was observed to release protoplasts on depletion of the substrate (2,12). The protoplasts were shown to be osmotically stable in sucrose (0.3 M), but could not be regenerated (12). During growth, *Methanosarcina mazei* characteristically undergoes a morphological change in which aggregates disperse releasing single, coccoid cells capable of forming new aggregates. Out studies have shown that single cells of strain S-6 are osmotically sensitive but are stabilized by sugars and divalent cations, and, in addition, electron microscopy reveals the absence of a cell wall. This species appears more promising for genetics since regeneration frequencies of 100% can be achieved in growth medium containing osmotic stabilizers.

Vectors. Plasmids are not known in mesophilic *Methanobacterium*, *Methanobrevibacter* and *Methanosarcina* species, which is due in part to the lack of a means of gently lysing the cells, although DNA extracted from protoplasts of *Methanosarcina* species has been examined. Bacteriophages have been observed by electron microscopy in growing cultures of *Methanobrevibacter smithii* strain PS suggesting that it is lysogenic. A sensitive host is being sought to aid the development of bacteriophage cloning vectors.

PROSPECTS AND CONCLUSIONS

The availability of selectable markers in hydrogenotrophic methanogens has made it possible to look for natural and artificial gene exchange, but at present the latter can only be attempted using intact cells and homologous linear chromosomal DNA. The release of viable single cells of *Methanosarcina mazei* has opened the door to genetic studies of the aggregate-forming acetotrophic methanogens; this species also offers the prospect of promoting genetic exchange and recombination by transformation and fusion of protoplasts once genetic markers have been obtained.

A further use for resistant mutants will be as marked strains with which to investigate the feasibility of 'seeding' digester populations during start-up, steady state operation or after digester failure. Efficient mutagenesis and selection techniques should also allow the isolation of strains with properties that are advantageous in the digester (Table 1).

Once gene transfer systems are developed, the 'target' genes for manipulation must be identified and isolated. Since mutations in the pathway for methanogenesis would be lethal to the cell, the genes involved may be isolated indirectly as previously reported (22) or directly by endogenous cloning, provided that suitable conditional lethal mutants can be obtained as recipients. *Methanosarcina* species are the most metabolically versatile methanogens, growing on hydrogen and carbon dioxide, acetate, methanol or methylamines and offer scope for investigating acetate utilisation.

As industrial micro-organisms for genetic engineering the methanogens present a unique challenge. Firstly, they combine the attributes of obligate anaerobes and archaebacteria with novel biochemical pathways; secondly, all strategies for genetic breeding must take into account the industrial habitat of methanogens, that is, a continuous mixed culture fermentation subject to fluctuating feed composition and loading rates. Genetically modified strains of methanogens must above all not be compromised in their ability to establish and maintain their numbers in the digester.

References

1   Archer, D.B. 1983. The microbiological basis of process control in methanogenic fermentation of soluble wastes. Enz. Microb. Technol. 5: 161-170.

2   Archer, D.B. and King, N.R. 1984. Isolation of gas vesicles from *Methanosarcina barkeri*. J. Gen. Microbiol. 130: 167-172.

3   Archer, D.B. and Harris, J.E. 1985. Methanogenic bacteria and methane production in various habitats. In: E.M. Barnes & G.C. Mead (eds.) Anaerobic bacteria in habitats other than man. pp.185-223. Society for Applied Bacteriology Symposium, Series 13. Blackwell Scientific Publications, Oxford.

4   Balch, W.E., Fox, G.E., Magrum, L.J., Woese, C.R. & Wolfe, R.S. 1979. Methanogens: reevaluation of a unique biological group. Microbiol. Reviews 43: 260-296.

5   Baresi, L. and Bertani, G. 1984. Isolation of a bacteriophage for a methanogenic bacterium. Abstracts Annual Meeting American Society for Microbiology I 74: p.133.

6   Beckler, G.5., Hook, L.A. and Reeve, J.N. 1984. Chloramphenicol acetyltransferase should not provide methanogens with resistance to chloramphenicol. Appl. Environ. Microbiol. 47: 868-869.

7   Bertani, G. and Baresi, L. 1984. Isolation of nutritional and other mutants in *Methanococcus voltae*. Abstracts Annual Meeting American Society for Microbiology I 73: p.133.

8   Bollschweiler, C. and Klein, A. 1982. Polypeptide synthesis in *Escherichia coli* directed by cloned *Methanobrevibacter arboriphilus* DNA. Zbl. Bakt. Microbiol. Hyg., I. Abt. Orig. C. 3: 101-109.

9   Bollschweiller, C., Kuhn, R. and Klein, A. 1985. Non repetitive AT-rich sequences are found in intergenic regions of *Methanococcus voltae* DNA. Embo. J. 4: 805-809.

10   Brown J.W. and Reeve J.N. 1985. Polyadenylated, non-capped RNA from the archaebacterium *Methanococcus vannielii*. J. Bacteriol. 162: 909-917.

11   Bryant, M.P. 1979. Microbial methane production - theoretical aspects. J. Animal Sci. 48: 193-201.

12   Davis, R.P. and Harris, J.E. 1985. Spontaneous protoplast formation by *Methanosarcina barkeri*. J. Gen. Microbiol. 131: 1481-1486.

13   Gujer, W. and Zehnder, A.J.B. 1983. Conversion processes in anaerobic digestion. Water Sci.Technol. 15: 127-167.

136

14   Hamilton, P.T. and Reeve, J.N. 1984. Cloning and
      expression of archaebacterial DNA from methanogens in
      Escherichia coli. In: W.R. Strohl & O.H. Tuovinen
      (eds.), Microbial Chemoautotrophy, The Ohio State
      University Press, Columbus, Ohio, U.S.A. p.291- 308.

15   Hamilton, P.T. and Reeve, J.N. 1985. Structure of
      genes and an insertion element in the methane
      producing archaebacterium *Methanobrevibacter smithii.*
      Mol. Gen. Genet. 200: 47-59.

16   Harris, J.E. and Pinn, P.A. 1985. Bacitracin-resistant
      mutants of   a mesophilic Methanobacterium species.
      Arch. Microbiol. (In press)

17   Jars, M., Altenbuchner, J. and Bock, A. 1983. Physical
      organization of the genes for ribosomal RNA in
      Methanococcus vannielii.
      Mol. Gen. Genet. 189: 41-47.

18   Jarsch, M. and Bock, A. 1983. DNA sequence of the
      16SrRNA/23SrRNA intercistronic spacer of two rDNA
      operons of the archaebacterium *Methanococcus
      vannielii.* Nucl.Acid Res. 11: 7537-7545.

19   Kaine, B.P., Gupta, R. and Woese, C.R. 1983. Putative
      introns in tRNA genes of prokaryotes.
      Proc. Natl. Acad. Sci. USA. 80: 3309- 3312.

20   Kiener, A., Holliger, C. and Leisinger, T. 1984.
      Analogue- resistant and auxotrophic mutants of
      Methanobacterium thermoautotrophicum.
      Arch. Microbiol. 139: 87-90.

21   Klein, A. and Schnorr, M. 1984. Genome complexity of
      methanogenic bacteria. J. Bacteriol. 158: 628-631.

22   Konheiser, U., Pasti, G., Bollschweiler, C. and Klein,
      A. 1984. Physical mapping of genes coding for two
      subunits of methyl CoM reductase component C of
      Methanococcus voltae. Mol. Gen. Genet. 198: 146-152.

23   Kronig, H., Semmler, R., Lerp, C. and Winter, J.
      1985. Evidence for the occurrence of autolytic
      enzymes in *Methanobacterium wolfei.*
      Arch. Microbiol. 141: 177-180.

24   Liu, Y., Boone, D.R., Sleat, R. and Mah, R.A. 1985.
      Methanosarcina mazei LYC, a new methanogenic isolate
      which produces a disaggregating enzyme.
      Appl. Environ. Microbiol. 49: 608-613.

25   Meile, L., Kiener, A. and Leisinger, T. 1983. A
      plasmid in the archaebacterium *Methanobacterium
      thermoautotrophicum.* Mol. Gen. Genet. 191: 480-484.

26   Meile, L. and Reeve, J.N. 1985. Potential shuttle
      vectors based on the methanogen plasmid pME2001.
      Bio/technology. 3: 69-72.

27   Mitchell, R.M., Loeblich, L.A., Klotz, L.C. and
      Loeblich, A.R. 1979. DNA organization of
      Methanobacterium thermoautotrophicum.
      Science. 204: 1082-1083.
28   Reeve, J.N., Trun, N.J. and Hamilton, P.T. 1982.
      Beginning genetics with methanogens In: A. Hollaender,
      R.D. DeMoss, S. Kaplin, J. Konisky, D. Savage and R.5.
      Wolfe (eds.), Genetic engineering of micro-organisms
      for chemicals. Plenum Press, New York, p.233-244.

29   Schmid G Pecher T. and Block A. 1982. Properties of
      the translational apparatus of Archaebacteria.
      Zbl. Bakt., Microbiol. Hyg., I. Abt. Orig. C. 3: 209-217.

30   Schmid, K., Thomm, M., Laminet, A., Laue, F.G.,
      Kessler, C., Stetter, K.O. and Schmitt, R. 1984. Three
      new restriction endonucleases Mae I, Mae II and Mae
      III from *Methanococcus aeolicus*.
      Nucleic Acid Res. 12: 2619-2628.

31   Thomm, A., Altenbuchner, J. and Stetter, K.O. 1983.
      Evidence for a plasmid in a methanogenic bacterium.
      J. Bacteriol. 153: 1060-1062.

32   Wich, G., Jarsch, M. and Bock, A. 1984. Apparent
      operon for a 5S ribosomal RNA gene and for tRNA genes
      in the archaebacterium *Methanococcus vannielii*.
      Mol. Gen. Genet. 196: 146-151.

33   Wood, A.G., Redborg, A.H., Cue, D.R., Whitman, W.B.
      and Konisky, J. 1983. Complementation of arg G and
      his A mutations of Escherichia coli by DNA cloned from
      the archaebacterium *Methanococcus voltae*.
      J. Bacteriol. 156: 19-29.

34   Zillig, W., Stetter, K.O., Schnabel, R., Madon, J.,
      Gierl, A. 1982. Transcription in archaebacteria.
      Zbl. Bakt., Microbiol. Hyg., I., Abt. Orig. C., 3: 218-227.

CHAPTER 13

GENETIC ANALYSIS OF TOXIN DETERMINANTS OF *CLOSTRIDIUM PERFRINGENS*

N.F. Fairweather, D.J. Pickard, P.M. Morrissey,
Valerie A. Lyness and G. Dougan.

Bacterial Genetics Group, Department of Molecular Biology,
Wellcome Biotechnology Ltd., Beckenham, Kent, U.K.

Contents

Introduction

Results

> Cloning of a haemolysin determinant from
> *C.perfringens* in *E. coli*.
>
> Subcloning of the haemolysin
> determinant into plasmid vectors.
>
> Analysis of the polypeptides expressed
> from the cloned haemolytic determinants.

Discussion

References

ABSTRACT

We have begun a genetic analysis of the toxins of *Clostridium perfringens*. A gene bank of *C. perfringens* type A strain CN1914 was constructed in *Escherichia coli* using the bacteriophage replacement vector lambda L47.1 . One hybrid phage, lambda WBL1, expressing a haemolysin was selected for further study. A 4.2 kb EcoRI fragment from lambda WBL1 was subcloned into the plasmid vector pACYC184 to give pCP100. Mutagenesis using the transposon Tn5 located the haemolysin gene to a 2.1 kb HindIII-EcoRI fragment, and this fragment was subcloned into the plasmid vector pUC8. The resultant plasmid, pCP101, expressed a protein of 49 000 daltons which cross-reacted immuno-logically with the streptolysin O of *Streptococcus pyogenes*. These results suggest that the gene encodes the theta toxin of *C. perfringens* although further work is required to confirm this.

The use of genetics as a tool to study the toxins of *C. perfringens* in greater detail is discussed. Genetics may allow a greater understanding of the mechanisms controlling expression of genes in the Clostridia and may enable greater exploitation of this genera in industrial and medical fields.

INTRODUCTION

C. perfringens strains produce at least twelve different toxins that may be involved in the pathogenesis of these organisms (4). Not all strains produce all twelve toxins and the production of the four major lethal toxins (alpha, beta epsilon and iota) is used to group the strains into five toxigenic types. Although in many cases there is a direct correlation between a disease and a particular toxigenic type, the role of many of the individual toxins in disease is unclear.

Genetic manipulation is an extremely useful tool which has been used to great effect to analyse the structure, regulation and expression of many proteins in a variety of species. It is now possible using recombinant DNA technology, to exploit genetics to characterise systems of regulation and expression in species where systems of gene transfer are ill characterised or non-existent. We have commenced a genetic analysis of the toxins in *C. perfringens* in order to study these toxins in greater detail including the regulation expression and their role in diseases associated with this species.

RESULTS

Cloning of a haemolysin determinant from *C. perfringens* in *E. coli*.

C. perfringens type A strain CN1914 was used as the source of target DNA. This strain produces at least two haemolytic toxins, alpha and beta, and possibly delta toxin, another haemolytic toxin. DNA was isolated and purified from this strain by lysing the cells according to the method of Hull et al. (2) and was partially cleaved with EcoRI to give fragments in the range 5-15 kilo-base pairs (kb). These fragments were ligated to DNA prepared from the replacement vector lambda L47.1, which had been completely cleaved with EcoRI, and the ligated products were packaged *in vitro* to generate intact phage particles. The packaged mixture was used to infect the *E. coli* host strain WL95 which carries a P2 prophage. Using this lysogenic strain, only recombinant phage can grow to generate plaques. About 10,000 independent recombinant plaques were pooled to generate a gene bank of *C.perfringens* DNA in *E. coli*.

The gene bank was then screened for the presence of phage expressing proteins with haemolytic activity as follows. Samples of the gene bank were plated out on *E.coli* C600 at a density of about 250 plaques per plate. After incubation overnight at 37°C the plates were overlayed with 1% (w/v) molten agarose in PBS containing 2.5% (v/v) packed washed rabbit erythrocytes. The plates were incubated at 37°C and after several hours large zones of haemolysis were seen around some of the plaques, occurring at a frequency of about one in every 700 plaques. One of these phage, lambda WBL1, was studied further.

Phage lambda WBL1 produced zones of haemolysis with sheep, horse or rabbit erythrocytes. This haemolysis was inhibited if cholesterol or a crude anti-theta toxin antiserum was included in the agarose overlay. The haemolysis was also inhibited by the addition of anti-streptolysin O serum. Streptolysin O is a cytolysin produced by group A Streptococci which displays immunological cross-reactivity with theta toxin (see reference 3). Both theta toxin and streptolysin O are inhibited by cholesterol. These results indicate that the recombinant phage WBL1 expresses a haemolysin which has the characteristics of the theta toxin of *C. perfringens*.

Subcloning of the haemolysin determinant into plasmid vectors.

DNA was prepared from lambda WBL1 and restriction enzyme digestion showed that this recombinant phage contained an insert of 14 kb which composed of three EcoRI fragments of

7.6, 4.2 and 2.4 kb. These three EcoRI fragments were cloned separately into the EcoRI site of plasmid vector pACYC184. Plasmid recombinants, harboured in the *E. coli* strain C600, were plated on agar containing sheep, rabbit or horse erythrocytes. Haemolytic zones were seen only with the plasmids containing the 4.2 kb fragment (figure 1) indicating that this fragment contains the determinant for haemolysin production.

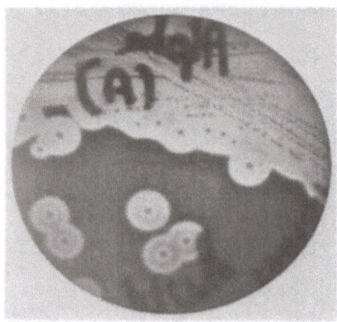

Figure 1. Haemolytic activity of *E. coli* harbouring plasmid pCP100. The strain was plated on sheep blood agar and incubated for 24 hours at 37°C.

One such plasmid, pCP100, was purified and a restriction map generated (see figure 2). The position of the haemolytic determinant within pCP100 was localised using Tn5 transposon mutagenesis. This technique involves the infection of cells harbouring a plasmid with a phage carrying the transposable element Tn5 encoding kanamycin resistance. Under the conditions used, the phage does not replicate in the cells and by selection for the antibiotic resistance, transposition of the resistance gene into the chromosomal and plasmid DNA occurs. The kanamycin resistant cells are pooled and plasmid DNA is prepared. This DNA is then transformed into fresh cells to give a population of cells each harbouring a plasmid containing the transposon. Cells transformed with pCP100 carrying the Tn5 transposon were plated out on agar containing

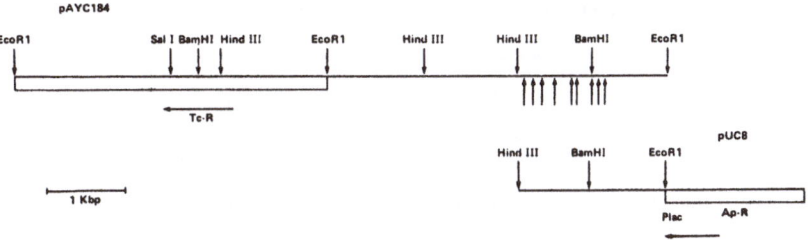

Figure 2. Physical map of plasmids pCP100 and pCP101. The open box represents the designated cloning vectors pACYC184 and pUC8 and the horizontal line represents sequences of the cloned *C.perfringens* DNA subcloned from lambda WBL1. Restriction enzyme sites are marked. The two horizontal arrows indicate the tetracycline resistance gene (Tc-R) of pACYC184 and the direction of transcription of lac promoter (Plac) present in pUC8. Ap-R designates the ampicillin resistance gene of pUC8. The vertical arrows indicate the approximate positions of the Tn5 insertions in the non-haemolytic pCP100-Tn5 plasmids described in the text.

rabbit erythrocytes and those colonies not giving zones of haemolysis were studied further. Plasmid DNA from twelve such colonies was analysed to locate the position of the transposon. Figure 2 shows that in each case the transposon mapped in a region of cloned DNA of about 1.3 kb which was located within a 2.1 kb HindIII-EcoRI fragment.

This fragment was subcloned into the plasmid vector pUC8 which had been cleaved with HindIII and EcoRI to generate the plasmid pCP101 (see fig. 2). Cells harbouring

pCP101 were strongly haemolytic when plated on blood agar
plates, haemolysis being detected several hours before
similar cells harbouring pCP100. This result indicates
that the gene encoding the haemolysin is located within
the 2.1 kb EcoRI- HindIII fragment.

Analysis of the polypeptides expressed from the cloned
haemolytic determinants. The polypeptides encoded by the
plasmids pCP100 and pCP101 were examined using the Western
blotting procedure. Total cell proteins of *E. coli* HB101
harbouring either pCP100 or pCP101 were separated by
sodium dodecyl sulphate-polyacrylamide gel electrophoresis
and the proteins transferred to nitrocellulose filters by
immunoblotting as described by Towbin *et al* (6). The
filters were then incubated with anti-strepyolysin O serum
followed by protein A conjugated to alkaline phosphatase.
A prominent band of 49,000 molecular weight was detected

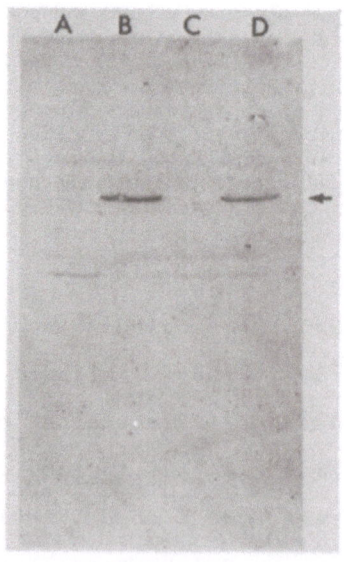

Figure 3. Western blot analysis of whole cell polypeptides after
separation on a 12.5% sodium dodecyl sulphate polyacrylamide gel.
Tracks are: (A) pACYC184; (B) pCP100; (C) pUC8; (D) pCP101. The
experiment was carried out as described in the text using anti-
streptolysin O antiserum. The arrow indicates the positions of the
immunoreactive proteins of 49,000 daltons in tracks B and D.

in the tracks harbouring proteins of cells containing pCP100 and pCP101, but not the vectors pACYC184 or pUC8 (figure 3).

DISCUSSION

We have used recombinant DNA technology to clone one genetic determinant of *C. perfringens* into *E.coli*. We constructed a gene bank using bacteriophage as a vector and we chose to screen for haemolytic determinants. This was in part due to the ease of screening for such a phenotype and also because *C. perfringens* produces at least two haemolytic toxins. The gene product we have analysed in this study has properties which strongly resemble those of theta toxin and it likely, although not definite, that we have cloned the gene for this toxin. Further experiments are necessary to confirm this. The haemolysis of the *E.coli* clones was inhibited by both cholesterol and a crude anti-theta serum both of which would be expected to inhibit theta toxin. Western blot analysis showed that cells containing the cloned gene expressed a protein of 49,000 daltons which reacted with anti streptolysin O serum. Theta toxin and streptolysin O are members of a group of immunologically and biochemically related oxygen labile haemolysins produced by different genera of Gram positive bacteria. The molecular weight of several of these haemolysins, including theta toxin, has been determined at around 60,000 daltons (3,4). Thus our estimate of a lower size of theta toxin may be an indication that we have cloned a different molecule that has properties similar to those of theta toxin. The analysis of several of these oxygen-labile toxins at the genetic level may throw some light on the structural relationships between these toxins.

The availability of cloned genes of *C. perfringens* is one requirement if we wish to study the regulation of expression of genes in *Clostridia*. Using our cloned DNA as a probe, it will be possible to probe DNA and RNA of various *C.perfringens* strains to ask whether all serotypes have the ability to express this gene. Thus if all strains have DNA which hybridises to the cloned DNA then the structural gene may be present but may not be expressed at high levels. Analysis of the RNA of these strains may reveal the extent of transcription of the genes in the various serotypes.

For a further study using genetics of *C. perfringens*, the other major requirements are a transformation system and a host-vector system. These have recently been described by Heefner et al (1) and Squires *et al* (5) and overcome some of the problems in studying the genetics of this species. It will therefore now be possible to introduce the toxin gene described above into *C. perfringens*. Because the gene would be on a multicopy plasmid, this approach would be expected to result in the production of large amounts of the toxin in *C. perfringens*. Squires *et al* have constructed 'shuttle vectors' which replicate in both *E. coli* and *C. perfringens*. It will be possible to manipulate the cloned *C. perfringens* DNA in *E. coli* to make specific alterations to the structural gene of the theta toxin. Thus if an antibiotic resistance gene were introduced into the theta toxin gene to render the gene inactive, this plasmid could then be reintroduced into *C. perfringens*. By forcing recombination with the host chromosome, the chromosomal gene encoding the haemolysin would be replaced by the mutated gene containing the antibiotic resistance determinant. Thus the *C.perfringens* strain would no longer produce theta toxin although the other toxins would still be produced. In this way, it will be possible to construct a series of strains which lack one of the many toxins of *C. perfringens*. The role of these toxins in disease may then be studied in appropriate animal models. In addition the isolation of the minor toxins could be made easier if this was carried out from strains which did not produce the major toxins which sometimes contaminate preparations of these molecules and so complicate their study.

References

1   Heefner,D.L., Squires,C.H., Evans,R.J., Kopp,B.J. and Yarus, M.J. 1984. Transformation of *Clostridium perfringens*. J. Bacteriol. 159: 460-464.

2   Hull, R.A., Gill, R.E., Hsu. P., Minshew, B.H. and Falkow, S. 1981. Construction and expression of recombinant plasmids encoding type 1 or d-mannose resistant pili from a urinary tract infection of an *Escherichia coli* isolate. Infect. Immun. 33: 933-938.

3   Kehoe, M. and Timmis, K.N. 1984. Cloning and expression in *Escherichia coli* of the Streptolysin O determinant from *Streptococcus pyogenes*: characterisation of the cloned streptolysin O determinant and demonstration of the absence of substantial homology with determinants of other thiol-activated toxins. Infect. Immun. 43: 804-810.

4   McDonel, J.L. 1980. *Clostridium perfringens* toxins (type A,B,C,D,E). Pharmac. Ther. 10: 617-655.

5   Squires, C.H., Heefner, D.L., Evans, R.J., Kopp, B.J. and Yarus, M.J. 1984. Shuttle plasmids for *Escherichia coli* and *Clostridium perfringens*. J. Bacteriol. 159: 465-471.

6   Towbin, H., Staehelin, T. and Gordon, J. 1979. Electrophoretic transfer of proteins from acrylamide gels to nitrocellulose sheets: procedures and applications. Proc. Natl. Acad. Sci. 76: 4350-4354.

CHAPTER 14

SULPHATE REDUCING BACTERIA AND THE OFFSHORE OIL INDUSTRY

W. A. Hamilton

Department of Microbiology, Marischal College, University of Aberdeen
Aberdeen, AB9 1AS

Contents

Abstract

Introduction

Corrosion

Sulphate-reducing bacterial growth and activity

Radiorespirometric assay

Conclusion

References

ABSTRACT

Corrosion is an electrochemical process. Microorganisms can influence the onset and development of corrosion either by assisting in the establishment of an electrolytic cell (indirect), or by stimulating the anodic or cathodic reactions (direct).

The presence, or absence of oxygen is a critical element in the mechanism of microbial corrosion. In the absence of oxygen the cathodic reaction involves the sulphate-reducing bacteria.

At the present time there are five separate hypotheses that seek to explain the mechanism of anaerobic microbial corrosion. The common thread running through each of these hypotheses is the central involvement of the metabolic activity of the sulphate-reducing bacteria; in particular the production of sulphide and the oxidation of hydrogen. The reason that there is as yet no clear consensus view as to the mechanism probably relates equally to two factors:- anaerobic microbial corrosion is inherently a complex process; experimental analyses have largely been carried out with pure cultures of sulphate-reducing bacteria.

The sulphate-reducing bacteria are found in nature as components of mixed microbial communities, or consortia which often exist as biofilms coating, for example, the surface of a steel pipe or offshore oil platform. The sulphate-reducing bacteria are dependent upon the other species within the consortium to supply their immediate nutrients (predominantly hydrogen and acetate), and to generate within an aerobic environment the anoxic conditions required for their metabolism and growth.

Appreciation of the importance of these aspects of the basic physiology and ecology of the sulphate-reducing bacteria is leading to the development of new experimental studies and, hopefully, new understanding of the mechanism of anaerobic microbial corrosion.

INTRODUCTION

The offshore oil and gas industries have three main centres of activity at the present time; the gas fields are principally located in the southern North Sea, with the major concentrations of oil being off Aberdeen (eg BP's Forties field) or north of Shetland (eg Shell's Brent and Chevron's Ninian fields). Production platforms are of two types; concrete gravity and steel jacket. Associated with the production, storage and transport of hydrocarbons on these platforms are a wide range of problems of microbial origin (Figure 1). These problems are of three general types. a) Corrosion can occur either externally on pipework and steel jacket platforms under marine fouling or discarded drill cuttings, or internally in water injection systems, oil risers, oil-water separators and in storage vessels, both offshore and onshore. b) A major problem can arise from the souring (i.e. an increase in the sulphide content of the produced hydrocarbons) or plugging of the reservoir. c) The production of sulphide within enclosed environments such as storage vessels and drilling legs on concrete platforms can cause severe problems for personnel safety. Major, although not the sole culprits in each of these problem areas are the sulphate-reducing bacteria.

In this paper I should like to concentrate on corrosion mechanisms and in particular on the role of the sulphate-reducing bacteria in these processes.

CORROSION

Microbial corrosion occurs by standard electrochemical mechanisms. The role of the microorganism is either to assist in the establishment of the electrolytic cell (indirect), or to stimulate the anodic or cathodic reactions (direct). Within the limits set by this broad statement it is possible to identify a number of detailed mechanisms and the involvement of various microbial species.

Corrosion, or rusting of material normally requires oxygen as the cathodic electron acceptor.

| Anodic reaction | $M \Longleftrightarrow M^{2+} + 2e$ |
| Cathodic reaction | $O_2 + H_2O + 4e \Longleftrightarrow 4OH^-$ |

Microbial slimes or tubercles from the aerobic growth of Pseudomonads or *Gallionella* respectively, can both generate oxygen concentration electrochemical cells (anodic at lower oxygen concentration beneath the growth or deposit) and supply oxygen as the cathodic reactant. Extensive corrosion occurs however in the complete absence of oxygen and such anaerobic corrosion is considered to be largely the consequence of the growth and activity of the sulphate-reducing bacteria.

There are at least five separately identifiable hypotheses for the mechanism of anaerobic microbial corrosion caused by sulphate-reducing bacteria. Firstly, the so-called classical cathodic depolarisation hypothesis proposes that the corrosion cell is under cathodic control with protons acting as electron acceptor and giving rise to atomic hydrogen. Although not mentioned in the original formulation of the hypothesis, an association reaction produces molecular hydrogen which can then be oxidised by hydrogenase-positive strains of sulphate-reducing bacteria

(22). While not totally discredited at the present time, this classical hypothesis is now seem as, at best, a partial or simplistic explanation.

Later hypotheses have placed considerable emphasis on the production of sulphide by the sulphate-reducing bacteria, and the development of iron sulphide films and deposits. King and Miller (8) proposed that the critical electrochemical reaction is the adsorption of the atomic hydrogen by the ferrous sulphide corrosion product, which is itself cathodic to the unreacted metal Ferrous sulphide is not however, a permanent cathode and its regeneration and the maintenance of a high and sustained corrosion rate is again dependent on the removal of this hydrogen by the action of bacterial hydrogenase.

Although Costello (1) also specified that the cathode is ferrous sulphide, he concluded that the cathodic reactant at neutral pH values is, in fact, hydrogen sulphide,

$$H_2S + e \Longleftrightarrow HS^- + \frac{1}{2} H .$$

Again hydrogenase may have an important, though secondary role through its removal of (molecular) hydrogen, with the further generation of more hydrogen sulphide.

Two other notable hypotheses of the mechanism of corrosion take very different views of the process. In a number of instances elemental sulphur has been noted in association with corrosion pits. It can be assumed that this may have arisen from the biotic or abiotic oxidation of sulphide at the aerobic/anaerobic interface. Sulphur is known to be highly corrosive and Schaschl (16) has proposed a concentration cell mechanism (analogous to an oxygen concentration cell under conditions of differential aeration) with the bacteria shielding the underlying metal (anode) from the higher concentration of dissolved sulphur

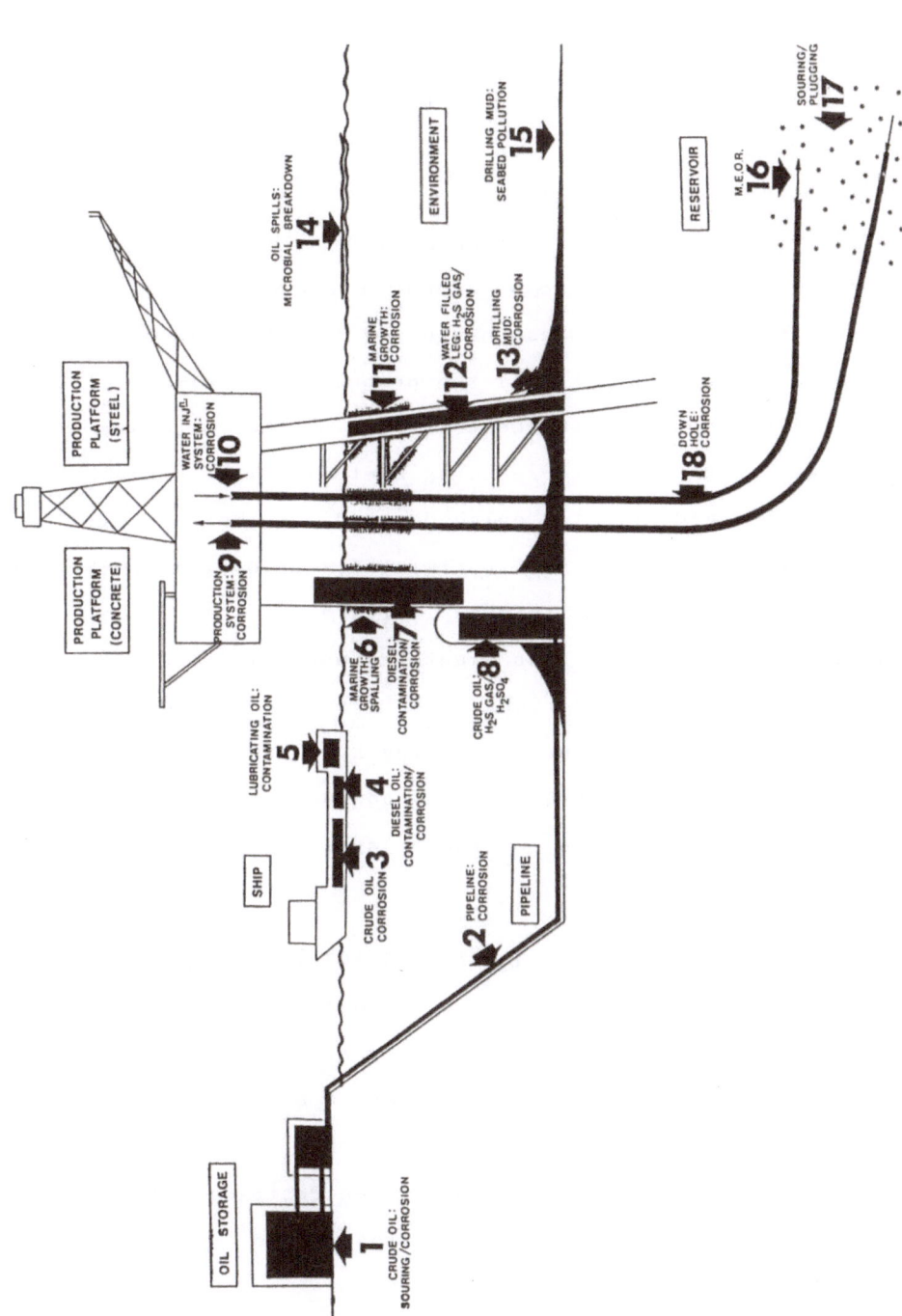

Figure 1. Impact of microorganisms on offshore oil and gas industries.

in the surrounding medium.

Mostly recently, Iverson (6) has formulated a corrosive metabolite hypothesis. The identity of the metabolite has still to be fully established but it appears to be phoshorous and volatile, in that cell contact is not necessary for metal corrosion to occur.

Fuller discussion of these mechanisms and of microbial corrosion in general is to be found in a number of review articles (4,9,12,21) and case histories (14,17,18,19).

The feature common to all the proposed mechanisms of anaerobic corrosion is the central role of the metabolic activities of the sulphate-reducing bacteria with respect to both the production of sulphide and, probably, the oxidation of hydrogen. Most experimental studies, however, have been carried out with pure cultures of sulphate-reducing bacteria in rich lactate-based media under controlled anaerobic conditions. The questions are how do such studies relate to our developing knowledge of this interesting group of bacteria, and how do they fit with our practical experience of those systems manifesting corrosion?

SULPHATE-REDUCING BACTERIAL GROWTH AND ACTIVITY

During the last 7 or 8 years our knowledge and understanding of the nutrition, physiology and ecology of the sulphate-reducing bacteria has undergone a major revision. Key figures in this development have been Widdel and Pfennig, Thauer and Peck, and Jorgensen Postgate and the present author have summarised the findings and discussed some of their implications.

We can now see that the sulphate-reducing bacteria are a relatively diverse group of bacteria which are related in terms of their cell physiology and their consequent ecological and economic impact. They are obligate anaerobes that use sulphate as alternative (to oxygen) electron acceptor with the resultant production of sulphide. Their carbon and energy nutrition is found not to be restricted to lactate and a few similar compounds, but to embrace a wide range of organics including fatty acids and in particular acetate (Table 1). The capacity to oxidise

Table 1. Newly identified species of sulphate-reducing bacteria

Species	Gram reaction Morphology	Nutrition		Electron Acceptor
1	— Curved rod	Fatty acids (C18)	----> Acetate Propionate	SO_4^{2-} ------>S^{2-}
2	— Lemon	Propionate	----> Acetate	SO_4^{2-} ------>S^{2-} NO_3^4 ------>NO_2^-
3	— Spore-forming rod	Acetate	----> CO_2	SO_4^{2-} ------>S^{2-}
4	— Rod	Acetate	----> CO_2	S^o ------>S^{2-}
5	— Rod to elliptical	Acetate	----> CO_2	SO_4^{2-} ------>S^{2-}
6	— Irregular in packages	Organic CO_2	----> CO_2 ----> Cell	SO_4^{2-} ------>S^{2-}
7	— Filaments (7 microns diameter)	Organic	------> CO_2	SO_4^{2-} ------>S^{2-}

1. *Desulfovibrio sapovarans*, 2. *Desulfobulbus propionicus*,
3. *Desulfotomaculum acetoxidans*, 4. *Desulfuromonas cetoxidans*,
5. *Desulfobacter postgatei*, 6. *Desulfosarcina variabilis*,
7. *Desulfonema magnum*

hydrogen as a source of energy for growth (acetate and CO supply the carbon) has been clearly documented and indeed hydrogen and acetate have been identified as principal nutrients in marine sediments. Sulphate-reducing bacteria are not found in isolation but in close physical and metabolic contact with other bacteria (or higher forms in the case of marine fouling). These communities of organisms are referred to as consortia; or biofilms where they occur on metal or other surfaces. Depending on the physical conditions prevailing and the primary nutrients available, microbial consortia may contain a wide range of aerobic, facultative and anaerobic organisms which together are capable of the hydrolytic and fermentative metabolism of primary nutrient sources such as carbohydrate, protein and other organic detritus, or hydrocarbons. The initial activities of the aerobic and facultative species will tend to utilise the available oxygen at a rate faster than it can be replaced by diffusion with the result that the innermost parts of the consortium will be anaerobic. It has variously been estimated that this effect is evident with biofilms of between 25 microns and 100 microns thickness. This leads to both the correct physicochemical conditions for the growth of sulphate-reducing bacteria and the continuous supply of their required nutrients, independent of the primary nutrient(s) supporting the growth of the biofilm as a whole (Figure 2). Additional hydrogen may also be available from the cathodic corrosion reaction. Clearly, the role of sulphate-reducing bacteria in such consortia which develop in sulphate-rich environments, parallels exactly that of methanogens in anaerobic digestors and the rumen.

RADIORESPIROMETRIC ASSAY

In respect, therefore, of the involvement of sulphate-reducing bacteria in corrosion processes it is only possible to get a meaningful measure of their *in situ* metabolic activity by studying the complete and undisturbed biofilm under conditions approximating as closely as

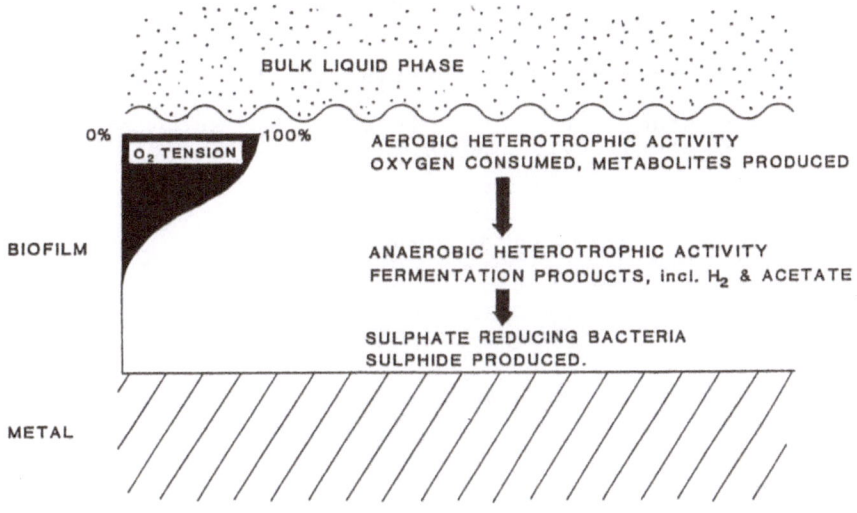

Figure 2.   Model for microbial biofilm.

possible to those prevailing in the corrosive environment.
This can very readily, and specifically, be done by a
[^{35}S] sulphate radiorespirometric assay.   Rosser and
Hamilton developed a simple test-tube technique suitable
for sediment analysis in the field.   We have now introduced a number of important modifications which have
proved necessary in adapting the technique to the study of
biofilms on the surface of metal corrosion coupons that
have been recovered after periods of exposure in
potentially corrosive environments (Figure 3).

Clearly this methodology has very considerable
potential in monitoring corrosion processes in the field,
determining biocide efficacy (5), and studying the
mechanism of corrosion.   Most notably, conditions have
been altered to make allowance for,

a) hydrogen gas evolution from the addition of acid to the metal coupon,

b) adsorption of [35S] sulphide on the rod and cup assembly,

c) saturation of the wick system with high levels of non-radioactive sulphide,

d) sulphate reduction occurring in sterile tubes,

e) inaccuracy at low levels of [35S] sulphate (eg. seawater) environments.

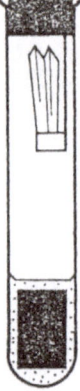

1. Metal coupon placed into 4 mls of anaerobic, filtered, sterile <u>sea water</u> containing <u>10 μCi</u> [35S—sulphate]

2. Bung seated securely and 0.5mls of oxygen-free 2N zinc acetate <u>immediately</u> injected onto the filter paper wick

3. Metal coupon incubated as desired temperature for <u>optimum incubation time</u> (in this case 5 hrs)

4. 0.5 mls of oxygen-free 6N hydrochloric acid injected passed the wick into the solution

5. Acid volatile sulphides, including any [H$_2$ ^{35}S] formed, trapped during a <u>2hr equilibration</u> period at 35 C, 100 osc. min^{-1} in a shaking water bath

(All manipulations carried out under oxygen-free nitrogen)

Fig. 3.   [35S] Radiorespirometric assay.

In the course of modifying the assay procedure, it was noted that maximal rates of [35S] turnover were achieved with shorter incubation times; 5hr being the chosen time for normal useage. Since it is possible that the apparently lower rate of activity during, for example, a 24hr incubation might be due to carbon limitation, this was tested directly using coupons which had been exposed in an estuarine environment for 66 days. Against controls with no added carbon source, test coupons were incubated with 34mM lactate or acetate (Figure 4). The stimulation evident in the 24hr incubations on the addition of both the sulphate-reducing bacteria in the biofilms are indeed carbon-limited, and that both lactate and acetate can meet

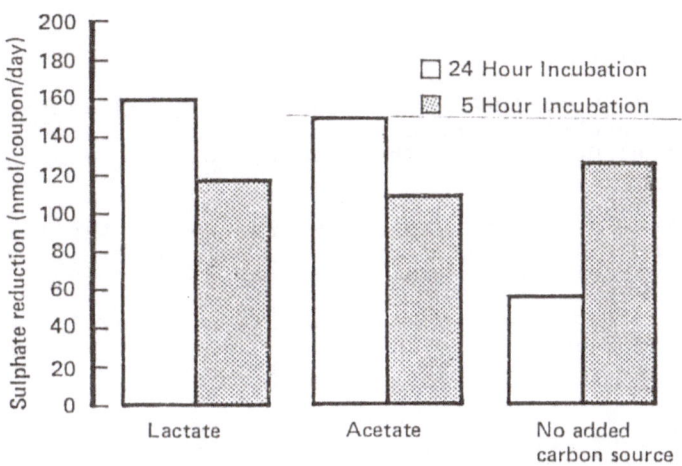

Fig. 4.   Stimulation of carbon-limited [35S] turnover.

carbon sources clearly shows that under these conditions that need and be oxidised with the reduction of more [35S] sulphate to sulphide.

CONCLUSION

While these data are still preliminary findings, they clearly demonstrate the relevance of the conceptual approach and the practical value of this methodology to the study of the mechanism and quantitative significance of sulphate-reducing bacteria in anaerobic microbial corrosion.

Acknowledgement

The author would like to express his appreciation of the support given to his laboratory by Shell U.K., British Petroleum and the Science and Engineering Research Council.

References

1   Costello, J.A. 1974. Cathodic depolarization by
     sulphate-reducing bacteria.
     South African J. Science. 70:   202-204.

2   Hamilton, W.A. 1983. Sulphate-reducing bacteria and
     the offshore oil industry.
     Trend. Biotechnol.1: 36-40.

3   Hamilton, W.A. 1983. The sulphate-reducing bacteria:
     their physiology and consequent ecology. In:
     Microbial Corrosion.   The Metals Society, London. pp
     1-5.

4   Hamilton, W.A. 1985. Sulphate-reducing bacteria and
     anaerobic corrosion.
     Ann. Rev. Microbiol. 39:   195-217.

5   Hardy, J.A. & Syrett, K.R. 1983. A radiorespirometric
     method for evaluating inhibitors of sulphate-reducing
     bacteria.   J. Appl. Microbiol. Biotechnol. 17:   47-52.

6   Iverson, W.P. 1984. Mechanism of anaerobic corrosion
     of steel by sulfate reducing bacteria.
     Materials Performance. 23 (3):   28-30.

7   Jorgensen, B.B. 1982. Ecology of the bacteria of the
     sulphur cycle with special reference to anoxic-oxic
     interface environments.
     Phil. Trans. R. Soc. Lond. B. 298:   543-561.

8   King, R.. and Miller J.D.A. 1971. Corrosion by the
     sulphate- reducing bacteria.   Nature. 233:   491-92.

9   Miller, J.D.A. 1971. In: Microbial Aspects of
     Metallurgy.   Medical and Technical Publishing Co.
     Ltd., Aylesbury. pp 1-202.

10   Odom, J.M. and Peck, H.D. 1984. Hydrogenase, electron
     transfer proteins and energy coupling in the sulfate-
     reducing bacteria Desulfovibrio.
     Ann. Rev. Microbiol. 38:   551-592

11   Pfennig, N., Widdel, F. and Truper H.G. 1981. The
     dissimilatory sulphate-reducing bacteria. In:M. P.
     Starr, H. Stolp, H.G.   Truper, A. Balows, H.G.
     Schlegel (ed.). The Prokaryotes.   Springer-Verlag,
     Berlin. pp. 926-940.

12   Pope, D.H., Duquette, D., Wayner, P.C. and Johannes,
     A.H. 1984.   In: Microbiologically Influenced
     Corrosion: A State-of-the Art Review. Materials
     Technology Institute of the Chemical Process
     Industries. Inc. Columbus, Ohio. pp. 1-76.

13   Postgate, J.R. 1984. In: The Sulphate-Reducing
     Bacteria. 2nd ed.   Cambridge Univ. Press. pp. 1-208.

14   Puckoris P.R. 1983. Massive utility condenser failure
     caused by sulfide producing bacteria.
     Materials Performance. 22 (12): 19-22.

15 Rosser, H.R. and Hamilton, W.A. 1983. Simple assay for accurate determination of [^{35}S] sulfate reduction activity. Appl. Environ. Microbiol. 45: 1956-1959

16 Schaschl, E. 1980. Elemental sulfur as a corrodent in deaerated, neutral aqueous solutions. Materials Performance. 19(7): 9-12.

17 Stoecker, J.G. 1984. Guide for the investigation of microbiologically induced corrosion. Materials Performance. 23(8): 48-55.

18 Tatnall, R.E. 1981. Case histories: bacteria induced corrosion. Materials Performance. 20(8): 41-8.

19 Tatnall, R.E. 1981. Fundamentals of bacteria induced corrosion. Materials Performance. 20(9): 32-8.

20 Thauer, R.K. 1982. Dissimilatory sulphate reduction with acetate as electron donor. Phil Trans. R. Soc. Lond. B. 298: 467-71.

21 Tiller A K 1982. Aspects of microbial corrosion. In: R.N. Parkins (ed.). Corrosion Processes. Appl. Sci. Publ., London and New York. pp 115-59.

22 von Wolzogen, C.A.H. and van der Vlugt, L.S. 1934. The graphitization of cast iron as an electrobiochemical process in anaerobic soils. Water (den Haag). 18: 147-65.

CHAPTER 15

PROSPECTS FOR THE GENETIC MANIPULATION OF RUMEN MICROORGANISMS

G.P. Hazlewood, S.P. Mann, C.G. Orpin and M.P.M. Romaniec

Department of Biochemistry, AFRC Institute of Animal Physiology, Babraham, Cambridge CB2 4AT, U.K.

Contents

Abstract

Introduction

Cloning of cellulase genes

Transfer of recombinant DNA to rumen bacteria

Plasmids of rumen bacteria

Conclusions

References

ABSTRACT

As the initial step in improving the rate and extent of ruminal cellulose breakdown through the use of recombinant DNA techniques, cellulase genes have been cloned from a cellulolytic rumen *Butyrivibrio* sp. and from *Clostridium thermocellum*. Transfer of recombinant DNA to rumen bacteria by transformation and conjugation has been investigated, and the distribution and size characteristics of plasmids in important genera of rumen bacteria have been evaluated. The probable benefits of fundamental genetic studies with rumen bacteria, to Agriculture and Industry are discussed.

INTRODUCTION

Ruminal fermentation of dietary material by a predominantly anaerobic microflora comprising bacteria (about 30 major species), ciliate protozoa (15 major species), flagellate protozoa and phycomycete fungi, is an essential step in the digestive process of the ruminant. In assessing the potential impact of biotechnology in farm animal production, it has been suggested that ruminant digestion could be beneficially altered if some characteristics of the fermentation were modified through the genetic manipulation of these rumen microorganisms (24). Detailed information in respect of genetic systems operating in the rumen anaerobic bacteria will be necessary for the application of recombinant DNA techniques, but the absence of such fundamental knowledge has not inhibited speculation regarding the potential of genetic engineering for improving the efficiency of animal production (1).

Domesticated ruminants occupy a prominent position in Agriculture because of their ability to convert plant products which are unfit for human consumption, to high quality animal protein, albeit at a low efficiency. Nevertheless, intensive beef and milk production currently depend on grain-based feeds. Future demands for animal products could be satisfied by feeding plant resources which are plentiful, cheap, renewable and not as usable for man, if the efficiency with which ruminants utilise diets high in cellulose and other insoluble carbohydrates can be improved (5). To this end, we are examining directly the feasibility of improving the rate and extent of cellulose breakdown in the rumen by using genetically-modified bacteria with enhanced cellulase activity. The many factors involved in obtaining expression of hetero-logous cellulase-encoding genes in a suitable recipient have recently been reviewed (23).

Genetic studies involving anaerobic bacteria in general and cellulolytic organisms in particular have implications both for Agriculture and for Industry. Only a small proportion of the millions of tonnes of crude fibre available is fed to animals; enormous potential exists for using the remainder as a substrate for solvent fermen-tations (6,17) or as animal feed after pretreatment with 'crude' cellulase produced by cloned cellulase genes from rumen microorganisms or after ensiling with agenetically-modified cellulolytic silage organism.

In other fundamental studies we are addressing some of the many problems (reviewed in reference 24) which currently preclude the application of conventional recom-binant DNA techniques to anaerobic rumen bacteria. The distribution and size characteristics of plasmids in some of the major genera of rumen bacteria have been evaluated, and work is in progress to reveal the phenotypes conferred by them and the identity of selectable markers. Hybrid plasmids incorporating a cryptic plasmid from a *Butyrivibrio* sp. and, in addition, indigenous plasmids are under examination as potential cloning vectors capable of replication in anaerobic rumen bacteria, as well as in bacteria with a well-characterised genetic system (*Escherichia coli*, *Bacillus subtilis*). Gene transfer mechanisms in anaerobic bacteria are also being investigated; these include naturally-occurring and induced transformation and conjugation.

In this paper we present an assessment of the progress made in genetic studies, with anaerobic bacteria, together with some of our own experimental results.

CLONING OF CELLULASE GENES

Cellulose comprises linear chains of β-1,4 linked glucose units, hydrogen-bonded to form highly-ordered crystalline entities (microfibrils) and requires the synergistic action of several enzymes to effect its complete hydrolysis to glucose: endo-1,4-β-D-glucanases which form free reducing chain ends and short-chain oligosaccharides by random cleavage of β-1,4 bonds in cellulose, exo-1,4-β-D-glucanases which form mainly cello-biose by endwise hydrolysis of the free reducing end of cellulose or cello-oligosaccharides and β-glucosidases which form glucose by endwise cleavage of cello-oligosaccharides. About 100 species of microorganisms are known to be cellu-lolytic (23) but detailed characterisation of cellulose-degrading enzymes has been reported for only about ten of them, including three species active in rumen cellulolysis, namely *Ruminococcus albus* (27,28), *Bacteroides succinogenes* (7,21) and *Ruminococcus flavefaciens* (19).

Possible mechanisms for enhancing rumen cellulolytic activity include amplification of cellulase genes in naturally-occurring bacteria, and the insertion of highly expressing heterologous cellulase genes into suitable recipient anaerobic bacteria. As source of cellulase genes for our studies we have selected two anaerobic bacteria: the first is a previously unstudied cellulolytic *Butyrivibrio* strain A46 which was isolated from the rumen of Svalbard reindeer (16), and grows vigorously in a medium containing acid-swollen cellulose as sole carbon source. The second is the anaerobic, cellulolytic, thermophile, *Clostridium thermocellum* NCIB 10682; the cellulase genes of this organism specify a complex but well characterised extracellular cellulolytic activity, capable of degrading crystalline cellulose (13, 18). They express well in different hosts, including *Saccharomyces cerevisiae* (20) and have been cloned and studied in *E.coli* (4). Using chromosomal DNA extracted from each of these

Table 1. Construction in *E.coli* of libraries containing cellulase genes.

Donor Organism	Vector	Cutting Enzyme for DNA	Ligation site in vector	Frequency of cellulase-positive clones[a]
Butyrivibrio A46	gtII	EcoRl	EcoRl	0.5
	pBR322	Pstl	Pstl	0
Clostridium	gtII	EcoRl	EcoRl	3.3
thermocellum	pBR322	Sau3A	BamHl	3.3
NCIB 10682	pHC79	Sau3A	BamHl	ND

[a] Frequency per thousand clones. At least 2,500 clones were screened. ND; not yet determined

organisms, and the procedures summarised in table 1, pseudo- random gene banks have been constructed in L phage and in *E. coli* HB101. DNA from *Butyrivibrio* A46, digested with EcoR1 and Pst1 has been cloned into phage vector Lambda gt11 and plasmid BR322, and that from *C.thermocellum* has been cloned in Lambda phage and also into the BamH1 sites of plasmid BR322 and cosmid HC79, after partial digestion with Sau3A. Cellulase-positive clones were identified by means of the Congo Red plate assay (26) which is based on the strong interaction between the dye Congo Red and polysaccharides containing more than 6 contiguous β-1,4- linked D-glucose units. Cellulase-positive *E. coli* clones (10) containing *C. thermocellum* DNA in plasmid BR322 were of two types (table 2), four (pRV1-4) producing large distinctive clear zones on carboxymethyl cellulose (CMC) plates and the remainder (pRV5-10) producing smaller, but nevertheless very definite zones. Cell-free extracts produced by brief sonication of *E.coli* clones pRV1-4 reduced the viscosity

Table 2. Characteristics of cellulase-positive *E. coli* clones containing *C. thermocellum* DNA in pBR322

			cell-free extracts	
Clone no.	Insert length (Kbp)	Congo Red plate assay halo diam.(mm)	Reducing sugar[a]	Viscometric assay[b]
pRV1	4.1	10	20.3	0.25
pRV2	2.6	8	10.8	0.48
pRV3	3.2	10	12.6	0.26
pRV4	4.2	10	13.8	0.25
pRV5	4.2	5	3.3	3.98
pRV6	5.0	4	2.9	4.03
pRV7	4.8	3	3.9	3.75
pRV8	4.3	4	4.5	2.93
pRV9	4.2	3	3.4	5.75
pRV10	5.5	4	2.2	9.75

[a] mcg glucose equivalent released.min^{-1}.(mg protein)$^{-1}$.
[b] time in hr. for 50% reduction in viscosity of CMC.

of CMC very rapidly (90% in <2h) and produced reducing sugar; extracts from clones pRV5-10 also attacked CMC reducing viscosity and producing a small yield of reducing end groups but much more slowly. On the basis of this evidence it is likely that each clone is expressing endo-β-1,4-glucanase activity; it is not apparent why clones pRV5-10 appear to express at a lower level, but it is interesting that genomic DNA from another cellulolytic rumen bacterium *B. succinogenes*, when cloned into *E. coli* using plasmid vector (pUC8), similarly gave rise to cellulase-positive clones with two levels of expression (3).

After restriction mapping and possibly subcloning, it is envisaged that cellulase genes will be inserted into a suitable vector and transferred to a rumen bacterium to test for expression of heterologous genes. To complement this approach, work has begun on the isolation and characterisation of regulatory sequences for highly expressed enzymes of *Butyrivibrio* sp. and *Streptococcus bovis*.

TRANSFER OF RECOMBINANT DNA TO RUMEN BACTERIA

The development of an *in vitro* system for transferring recombinant DNA to suitable recipient anaerobes is an essential step in determining whether rumen bacteria can be modified through the insertion and expression of heterologous genes. Possible DNA transfer mechanisms are transformation, conjugation and transduction; potential vectors include previously-described broad host range plasmids, indigenous plasmids, and hybrid plasmids (shuttle vectors) containing replication origins from at least two different species and able to replicate in a well-characterised genetic system (*E. coli*, *B. subtilis*).

To test for natural transformation in the genus *Butyrivibrio*, we have attempted to convert the general fatty acid auxotroph, *Butyrivibrio* S29 to prototrophy by transforming with chromosomal DNA extracted from 6 wild-type strains of *B. fibrisolvens*. Mid-log phase cells of the auxotrophic recipient were treated with wild-type DNA at two different temperatures (39° C and 0° C) and transformants were selected for in both solid and liquid restrictive medium, deficient in long-chain fatty acid, but otherwise complete. In two experiments, no transformants were recovered, and it is uncertain at this stage whether this is solely due to the failure of the recipient cells to develop competence.

Where natural competence does not occur, artificially-induced transformation has been achieved by $CaCl_2$ treatment, osmotic shock, freezing and thawing, growth in hypertonic medium and penicillin treatment (12). With the exception of $CaCl_2$ treatment of *E.coli* cells (14), PEG-induced uptake of plasmid DNA by protoplasts followed by regeneration of the cell wall and selection of transformants, is the most efficient method of artificially-induced transformation (12).

Plasmid transformation of anaerobic bacteria has only been reported in *C. perfringens* and was achieved by the use of an L-phase variant (10). Unlike protoplasts, L-phase or wall-less cells will grow and divide in liquid medium, so phenotypic expression and selection of transformants can occur without the need to establish the sometimes rigorous conditions necessary to promote cell wall regeneration at a reasonable frequency.

To facilitate our attempts at transforming rumen bacteria, conditions have been established for quantitatively converting *Butyrivibrio* spp. (strains Bu49 and PI-7) to protoplasts (8), and promoting regeneration of the cell wall, albeit at a low frequency. In addition, protoplasts of strain PI-7 cells grown in rich medium were converted to osmotically-fragile L-phase cells if plated in a soft agar overlay on rich medium and subsequently transferred in an agar plug to liquid medium containing 15% (w/v) sucrose and penicillin (200 mcg/ml). The procedure of Chang and Cohen (2), adapted to allow the use of anaerobic buffers and strictly anaerobic handling procedures, has been used in experiments to transfer a variety of broad host range plasmids, expressing selectable antibiotic resistances in both Gram-negative and Gram-positive cells, to protoplasts and L-phase cells of the two butyrivibrios, but to date, no stable transformants have been detected in either solid or liquid selective media. In separate experiments, kanamycin resistance of pUB110 and chloramphenicol resistance of pRK2 were apparently transferred to L-phase cells and protoplasts of strain PI-7 respectively, but were lost on subculture. To examine the possibility that artificially-induced transformation with broad host range plasmids failed because of the absence of replication origins that function in rumen *Butyrivibrio* spp., we have constructed a series of shuttle plasmids containing a 2.8 Kbp cryptic plasmid from *Butyrivibrio* sp. strain Bu49 ligated to the *E. coli* plasmids pAT153 and pBR325 and the *E. coli / B. subtilis* shuttle vector pHV33 (table 3) (15). Each of the hybrid plasmids was transformed into CaCl$_2$-treated *E. coli* and was stably maintained, but PEG-induced transformation of L-phase cells of Butyrivibrio strain PI-7 and protoplasts of plasmid-free strain Bu49 has not been successful. In addition to transformation, we have examined conjugation as a means of transferring plasmid-borne functions to recipient rumen bacteria from *E. coli* strains containing broad host range conjugative plasmids. Log phase cells of randomly-isolated butyrivibrios (10 strains), selenomonads

Table 3. Construction of *E. coli/B. fibrisolvens* hybrid plasmids

| | Designation | | | |
	pOM41	pOM62	pOM121	pOM221
Size (Kbp)	8.8	8.6	7.5	9.7
Parent plasmid designation	pBR325	pBR325	pAT153	pHV33
size (Kbp)	6.0	6.0	3.6	6.9
markers	Ap^r Cm^r Tc^r	Ap^r Cm^r Tc^r	Ap^r Tc^r	Ap^r Cm^r Tc^r
site used	EcoR1	Pst1	Pst1	Pst1
Phenotype of *E. coli* transformation[b]	Ap^r Cm^s Tc^r	Pp^s Cm^r Tc^r	Ap^s Tc^r	Ap^s Cm^r Tc^r

[a] Comprises *B. fibrisolvens* cryptic plasmid, pOM1 (2.8 Kbp) and an *E. coli* plasmid.
[b] after transformation with hybrid plasmid.

(6 strains) and total mixed rumen bacteria were mixed under anaerobiosis with *E. coli* strains containing pRI, pRK2, pRPI, pRP4 and pRK404 (the latter mobilised in a triparental mating with the self-transmissible helper plasmid pRK2013) and were plated on filters or directly onto medium containing cellobiose as carbon source and streptomycin (200 mcg/ml), both of which counter-selected against the donor. Transconjugants were selected on medium containing tetracycline (5 mcg/ml) or chloramphenicol (20 mcg/ml). No evidence was obtained for the transfer of conjugative plasmids to butyrivibrios or selenomonads, but an apparent transconjugant with the Tcr phenotype was

generated when *E. coli* bearing pRPI was mated with mixed rumen bacteria. The organism, which was a Gram-negative non-motile fusiform rod, did not arise spontaneously on control plates and contained a single plasmid of around 10 Kbp which may have resulted from the extensive deletion of non-essential regions of pRPI; such a phenomenon has been previously reported for the large IncP incompatibility group plasmids RPI/RP4/RK2 (22).

PLASMIDS OF RUMEN BACTERIA

The general characteristics of the rumen environment seem likely to promote the development of plasmid-borne functions, yet, with the exception of some bovine strains of *Butyrivibrio fibrisolvens* which are reported to contain a large (250 megadalton) cryptic plasmid (25), plasmids have not been described in anaerobic rumen bacteria.

Our own studies in this area are directed at establishing the distribution and size characteristics of rumen plasmids and the phenotypes conferred by them. Using a rapid plasmid screening method (11), a systematic survey of 90 butyrivibrios isolated at random from five Svalbard reindeer in an intermixing herd (16), revealed that 24 strains from three different animals contained one or more plasmids in the approximate size range 2-4 Kbp; two further bovine isolates including strain Bu49 which contained the 2.8 Kbp plasmid, pOM1, used in constructing the previously described shuttle vectors, were found to have plasmids.

Sixty-five percent of selenomonads isolated at random from goat and cow rumen contents on a medium with glucose as carbon source contained one or more plasmids and all strains isolated on media containing either lactate (*S.ruminantium* var. *lactilytica*) or xylose as sole carbon source contained plasmids. Some strains carried up to six plasmids and approximate sizes varied from less than 3 Kbp to greater than 24 Kbp. Further experiments with selenomonads have indicated a positive correlation between carbon compounds fermented and the presence of certain plasmids.

Plasmids of about 8 Kbp and greater than 24 Kbp have been found in different strains of *S. bovis* but the proportion of strains with plasmids remains uncertain.

CONCLUSIONS

Modification of rumen function through the application of recombinant DNA techniques will clearly require a great deal of research, not least because so little is known about the genetic systems operating in rumen bacteria. Cellulase genes from cellulolytic anaerobes have been successfully cloned and partially characterised. Due to deficiencies in either the transfer mechanism or the plasmid vectors selected for use, a routine procedure for transferring the recombinant DNA to rumen bacteria has not yet been established. Nevertheless, the detection of unstable recombinants in some of our experiments is promising. Once the identity of selectable marker genes has been established, indigenous plasmids may have the potential to solve this problem. Because of current interest in using anaerobic bacteria in fermentation processes for converting cheap, renewable, plant resources or cellulosic wastes to valuable products (e.g. biofuels, solvents), it seems possible that the cloned genes of rumen bacteria, especially those coding for cellulases, will have more immediate uses in Industry.

References

1   Armstrong , D.G. 1985.   The potential of
     biotechnology for the improvement in farm livestock
     production.   In: The Feed Compounder 5: 16-19.

2   Chang, S. and Cohen, S.N. 1979. High frequency
     transformation of *Bacillus subtilis* protoplasts by
     plasmid DNA.   Molec. Gen. Genet. 168: 111-115.

3   Crosby, B., Collier, B., Thomas, D.Y., Teather, R.M.
     and Erfle, J.D., 1984.   Cloning and expression in
     Escherichia coli of cellulase genes from *Bacteroides
     succinogenes*.   In: S. Hasnain (ed.).   Proceedings of
     Fifth Canadian Bioenergy R. and D. seminar.
     Elsevier. pp. 573-576.

4   Cornet, P., Millet, J., Beguin, P. and Aubert, J.P.
     1983.   Characterization of two cel (cellulose
     degradation) genes of *Clostridium thermocellum* coding
     for endoglucanases.   Biotechnol. 1: 589-594.

5   Engelhardt, W.V., Dellow, D.W. and Hoeller, H.   1985.
     The potential of ruminants for the utilization of
     fibrous low-quality diets.   Proc. Nutr. Soc. 44: 37-43.

6   Eveleigh, D.E. 1981.   The microbiological production
     of industrial chemicals.   Scient. Am. 245: 120-130.

7   Groleau, D. and Forsberg, C.W. 1983.   Partial
     characterisation of the extracellular endoglucanase
     produced by *Bacteroides succinogenes*.
     Can. J. Microbiol. 29: 504-517.

8   Hazlewood, G.P., Cho, K.Y., Dawson, R.M.C. and Munn,
     E.A. 1983.   Subcellular fractionation of the Gram
     negative rumen bacterium, *Butyrivibrio* S2, by
     protoplast formation, and localisation of lipolytic
     enzymes in the plasma membrane.
     J. Appl. Bacteriol. 55: 337-347.

9   Hazlewood, G. and Dawson, R.M.C.   1979,
     Characteristics of a lypolytic and fatty acid-
     requiring *Butyrivibrio* sp. isolated from the ovine
     rumen.   J. Gen. Microbiol. 112: 15-27.

10   Heefner, D.L., Squires, C.H., Evans, R.J., Kopp, B.J.
     and Yarus, M.J. 1984.   Transformation of *Clostridium
     perfringens*.   J. Bacteriol. 159: 460-464.

11   Kieser, T. 1984.   Factors affecting the isolation of
     CCC DNA from *Streptomyces lividans* and *Escherichia
     coli*.   Plasmid 12: 19-36.

12   Klebe, R.J., Harriss, J.V., Sharp, Z.D. and Douglas,
     M.G. 1983.   A general method for polyethylene-glycol-
     induced genetic transformation of bacteria and
     yeasts.   Gene 25: 333-341.

13   Lamed, R., Kenig, R., Setter, E. and Bayer, E.A.
      1985. Major characteristics of the cellulolytic
      system of *Clostridium thermocellum* coincide with
      those of the purified cellulosome.
      Enzyme Microb. Technol. 7: 37-41.

14   Maniatis, T., Fritsch, E.F. and Sambrook, J. 1982.
      Molecular Cloning, A laboratory manual. Cold Spring
      Harbor Laboratory, Cold Spring Harbor, N.Y.

15   Mann, S.P., Hazlewood, G.P. and Orpin, C.G. 1985.
      Characterisation of a cryptic plasmid (pOM1) in
      Butyrivibrio fibrisolvens by restriction
      endonuclease analysis and its cloning in *Escherichia
      coli*. Curr. Microbiol.: submitted.

16   Orpin, C.G., Mathiesen, S.D., Greenwood, Y. and Blix,
      A.S. 1985. Seasonal changes in the ruminal
      microflora of the High-Arctic Svalbard Reindeer
      (Rangifer Tarandus Platyrhynchus).
      Appl. Environ. Microbiol.: accepted.

17   Payton, M.A. 1984. Production of ethanol by
      thermophilic bacteria. Trends Biotechnol. 2: 153-158.

18   Petre, J., Longin, R. and Millet, J. 1981.
      Purification and properties of an endo-β-1,4-
      glucanase from *Clostridium thermocellum*.
      Biochimie (Paris) 63: 629-639.

19   Pettipher, G.L. and Latham, M.J. 1979.
      Characteristics of enzymes produced by *Ruminococcus
      flavefaciens* which degrade plant cell walls.
      J. Gen. Microbiol. 110: 21-27.

20   Sacco, M., Millet, J. and Aubert, J.P. 1984. Cloning
      and expression in *Saccharomyces cerevisiae* of a
      cellulase gene from *Clostridium thermocellum*.
      Ann. Microbiol. (Paris) 135A: 485-488.

21   Schellhorn, H.E. and Forsberg, C.W. 1984.
      Multiplicity of extracellular β-(1,4)-endoglucanases
      of *Bacteroides succinogenes* S85.
      Can. J. Microbiol. 30: 930-937.

22   Schwab, H., Saurugger, P.N. and Lafferty, R.M. 1983.
      Occurrence of deletion plasmids at high rates after
      conjugative transfer of the plasmids RP4 and RK2
      from *Escherichia coli* to *Alcaligenes eutrophus* H16.
      Arch. Microbiol. 136: 140-146.

23   Seligy, V.L., Barbier, J.L., Dimock, K.D., Dove,
      M.J., Moranelli, F., Morosoli, R., Willick, G.E. and
      Yaguchi, M. 1983. Current status in the application
      of recombinant DNA technology in the construction
      of cellulolytic yeast strains. In: M. Korhola and
      E. Vaisanen (ed.). Gene expression in yeast.
      Proceedings of the Alko yeast symposium, Helsinki.
      pp. 167-185.

24   Smith, C.J. and Hespell, R.B. 1983. Prospects for
      development and use of recombinant deoxyribonucleic
      acid techniques with ruminal bacteria.   J. Dairy
      Sci. 66: 1536-1546.

25   Teather, R.M. 1982. Isolation of plasmid DNA from
      Butyrivibrio fibrisolvens.
      Appl. Environ. Microbiol. 43: 298-302.

26   Teather, R.M. and Wood, P.J.   1982.   Use of
      Congo Red-polysaccharide interactions in enumeration
      and characterization of cellulolytic bacteria from
      the bovine rumen.   Appl. Environ. Microbiol. 43: 777-780.

27   Wood, T.M. and Wilson, C.A. 1984. Some properties of
      the endo-(1 -> 4-β-D-glucanase synthesized by the
      anaerobic cellulolytic rumen bacterium *Ruminococcus
      albus*.   Can. J. Microbiol. 30: 316-321.

28   Wood, T.M., Wilson, C.A. and Stewart, C.S. 1982.
      Preparation of the cellulase from the cellulolytic
      anaerobic rumen bacterium *Ruminococcus albus* and its
      release from the bacterial cell wall.
      Biochem. J.   205: 129-137.

CHAPTER 16

COMMERCIAL EXPLOITATION OF CELLULOLYTIC ANAEROBES

R. Sleat

Biotechnica Ltd., 5 Chitern Close, Llanishen, CARDIFF, CF4 5DL

Contents

Abstract

Introduction

Cellulose and cellulases

    Exoglucanase activity

    Endogluconase activity

    β-glucosidase

Cellulases from strictly anaerobic microorganisms

Chemical and fuel production by cellulolytic anaerobes

    Indirect

    Direct

    Coupled

        a. Two-membered culture fermentation

        b. Multi-component fermentation

Conclusions

References

ABSTRACT

There is increasing recognition of, and interest in, the possibility of using renewable lignocellulosic materials as feedstocks for the production of chemicals and fuels. Both chemical and biological means exist for the hydrolysis of the cellulose fraction of lignocelluloses. Anaerobic microbial hydrolysis of cellulose and subsequent fermentation of released sugars result in high recoveries of the carbon and energy in the substrate as potentially useful endproducts. Anaerobic cellulolytic bacteria may play an important role in the commercial exploitation of lignocellulosic materials. Advances in our understanding of the ecology, physiology and biochemistry of these microorganisms will ensure the efficient utilization of cellulose. The production of fuels and chemicals from renewable resources will do much to decrease society's dependence on petroleum and petroleum-based products.

INTRODUCTION

The production of industrially important chemicals by microbial fermentations is not a new concept. Acetone and butanol production by *Clostridium acetobutylicum* was of great importance in the manufacture of explosives and aeroplane wing dope during the first world war. The "fuel crisis" of the early seventies saw much effort directed towards the production by microbial action of the non-petroleum based fuels ethanol and methane from agricultural, industrial and municipal wastes. Ethanol and methane, derived from anaerobic fermentations of renewable biomass,

offered possible alternatives to petroleum fuels.
Industrially important chemicals and fuels produced by
anaerobic fermentations are becoming increasingly viable
economic alternatives to conventional petroleum-dependent
products. This has arisen as a result of a number of
factors, amongst which some of the most important are: a
realization of the need to preserve valuable, finite
petroleum resources for the production of chemicals that
cannot be made economically by alternative means;
increasing political and environmental pressure to find
less energy-intensive methods of disposing of agricultural,
industrial and municipal wastes; larger government and EEC
subsidies as incentives for examining alternative means of
saving fuel resources; the potential for using renewable
biomass as fermentation feedstocks for the production of
chemicals of industrial importance; greater understanding
of the microbiology and biochemistry of fermentation
systems, which has resulted in increasing yields of
compounds of interest;, developments in the field of downstream processing which enable more efficient recovery of
fermentation products.

Chemical and fuel production by anaerobic bacteria is
the subject of an excellent review by Zeikus (33). In
this short paper, I will concentrate on the role that
cellulose, anaerobic cellulolytic bacteria and cellulases
may play in industrial processes.

CELLULOSE AND CELLULASES

Cellulose-containing materials have been broadly
divided into three categories (5). Primary cellulosics
were defined as those cellulosics which are produced for
their cellulose, structural or food content. The second

group, agricultural waste cellulosics, includes all those cellulosics which arise from the harvesting and processing of agricultural material. Animal manures are included in this group. The final category comprises the municipal waste cellulosics. The production of waste cellulosics in the UK is shown in Table 1. Tremendous quantities of waste cellulose-containing waste material are generated

Table 1. Production of primary and waste cellulosics in the United Kingdom

Material	Year	Annual Production (tonnes x 10^{-6})	Cellulose content (%)
Timber	1983-4		
Total cut		5.5	45
Harvested		4.2	
Waste		1.3	
Hay	1982	6.6	35
Animal manures	1984		15
Total		120	
Housed livestock		70	
Cereal straws	1984		42-49
Total		17.8	
Baled		10.2	
Burnt		6.3	
Soil incorporated		1.2	
Waste to landfill	1983	20	32-37

Sources: Forestry Commission Facts and Figures 1983-4; Farm waste management unit, Ministry of agriculture, fisheries and food; Dr. S.B.C. Larkin Dept. of Agricultural Engineering, Silsoe College, Silsoe, Bedford; Dr. J.F. Rees, Biotechnica Ltd., Cardiff.

annually in the U.K. The most significant, in terms of weight, is that derived from animal manures. Its potential as a feedstock for chemical production may be limited, but its value as a substrate for methane production has long been recognized (9). The most significant source of cellulosic wastes is the paper-basedproducts found in municipal refuse. This material is cheap and methods of collection and storage are well established. Methane generated from municipal refuse disposed to landfills is an important commodity which is being commercially exploited at a number of sites in the U.K., Europe and the U.S.A. Both physical and chemical methods have been developed to increase the value of municipal refuse as a feedstock for methane production (16). Cereal straws represent a large reserve of cellulose-containing material. Legislation may soon be strengthened to prohibit the burning of straws in fields and alternative means of disposal are being sought. The possibility of producing fuel gas from agricultural crop residues has been investigated (30).

Cellulose is a linear polymer of anhydroglucose molecules connected through β -(1-4)-glycosidic linkages. Elementary cellulose microfibrils comprise highly ordered bundles of cellulose chains with interspersed amorphous regions. In plants, cellulose is found in both the primary and secondary cell walls. The physical structure of cellulose and its degree of association with the poly-aromatic macromolecule, lignin, affect the rate of bio-degradation. Biological cellulose degradation results from the transformation of a molecule with a high degree of polymerization ($<=15,000$) into small molecular weight oligosaccharides which are further converted to the disaccharide, cellobiose, and glucose. This process can be viewed as a biological hydrolysis. Chemical methods have been developed for the hydrolysis of cellulose into its component monomers (13) but these methods will not be discussed further here. Biological degradation is accomplished by a group of enzymes generically termed cellulases. Three major components have been identified in cellulases which are important in complete saccharification of native cellulose.

Exoglucanase activity. 1,4-β-D-glucan cellobiohydrolase
(EC. 3.2.1.91). Exoglucanase removes cellobiose or,
rarely, glucose from the non-reducing ends of cellulose
molecules.

Endoglucanase activity. 1,4-β-D-glucan 4-glucanohydrolase
(EC. 3.2.1.4.). Endoglucanase hydrolyzes β-1,4 glycosidic
linkages randomly along the cellulose molecule.

Beta-Glucosidase. β-D-glucoside glucohydrolase (EC.
3.2.1.21). β-glucosidase removes glucose from the non-
reducing ends of both cellobiose and small chain oligosaccharides. Activity decreases with increasing chain
length of the cellodextrins.

Complete saccharification of cellulose requires the
synergistic action of all three cellulase components.
Endoglucanase acts upon the amorphous regions of cellulose.
This results in the production of new non-reducing chain
ends. Exoglucanase activity sequentially removes
cellobiose moieties from these ends. This results in the
eventual breakdown of the crystalline portion of the
molecule and generates amorphous regions susceptible to
endoglucanase activity. β-glucosidase complements these
activities by removing cellobiose, a potential end-product
inhibitor of exo- and endoglucanase, from the hydrolysis
system.

Commercial exploitation of cellulose by strictly
anaerobic cellulolytic bacteria requires complete saccharification into cellobiose or preferably glucose. If
cellulases derived from strict anaerobes are to be compe-
titive with fungal cellulases as a means of hydrolyzing
cellulose a number of criteria have to be met: the
possession of all three component activities, high

stability, high specific activity and efficient production of cellulase in commercial quantities. Some of these requirements are now being addressed.

CELLULASES FROM STRICTLY ANAEROBIC MICROORGANISMS

Strictly anaerobic microorganisms capable of cellulose degradation have been listed in Table 2. The renewed

Table 2. Strictly anaerobic cellulose degrading microorganisms.

Microorganism	Source
Bacteroides succinogenes *Butyrivibrio fibrisolvens* *Ruminococcus albus* *Ruminococcus flavefaciens* *Eubacterium cellulosolvens* *Clostridium cellobioparum* *Clostridium longisporum* *Clostridium lochheadii* *Neocallimastix frontalis*	Rumen
Bacteroides cellulosolvens *Clostridium thermocellum* *Acetivibrio cellulolyticum* *Acetivibrio cellulosolvens* *Clostridium cellulovorans* *Clostridium populeti*	Digesters
Clostridium cellulolyticum	Decaying grass
Clostridium papyrosolvens	Estuarine sediments
Clostridium stercorarium	Manure
Clostridium sp.	Freshwater sediments
Bacteroides sp.	Human faeces
Bacteroides succinogenes *Ruminococcus flavefaciens*	Rat caecum

interest in cellulose decomposition by strict anaerobes is reflected in the numbers of these species that have been isolated in the last few years. The list includes the first reported strictly anaerobic fungus, *Neocallimastix frontalis* (20). *Clostridium longisporum* and *Clostridium lochheadii* were isolated by Hungate (10) in the fifties but have rarely been observed since. However, *Clostridium cellulovorans* (27) resembles *C.lochheadii* in many respects.

The exo-and endoglucanase activities of commercial cellulases are compared in Table 3 with those of cellulases from a number of anaerobic bacteria. The cellulases from strict anaerobes are oxygen tolerant although activity is enhanced by reducing agents (15,15,25,32). Exo- and endoglucanse activities are present in *A. cellulolyticus*, *C. thermocellum* and *C. cellulovorans*. Exoglucanase is generally determined by its ability to release reducing sugars from the microcrystalline cellulose substrate, Avicel. Judging from this assay procedure, *N. frontalis* apparently possesses very little exoglucanase activity. Mountfort and Asher (15) determined that activity towards long-chain oligosaccharides by *N. frontalis* culture supernatant was six-fold higher

Table 3. Activities of commercial cellulases and cellulases from anaerobic microorganisms.

Microorganism	Exoglucanase activity	Endoglucanase	Ref
B. succinogenes	−	+	7
R. flavefaciens	+	−	24
R. albus	−	+	32
N. frontalis	+/−	+	15
A. cellulolyticus	+	+	25
C. thermocellum	+	+	17
*C. cellulovorans**	+	+	
C. cellulolyticum	+/−	+	6
Penicillium funiculosum (Sigma)	+ +		
Aspergillus niger (Sigma)	−	+	
Trichoderma viride (Sigma)	−	+	
Trichoderma viride (BDH)	−	+	

* unpublished results

than that for Avicel. They concluded that oligosaccharide was a better substrate for the determination of exoglucanase activity. The presence of exoglucanase is not an absolute prerequisite for the complete saccharification of microcrystalline cellulose. *B. succinogenes* (7) and *R. albus* (32) cultures both actively degrade Avicel whilst cell-free culture supernatants do not. Wood and Wilson (32) have suggested that either "a localized high concentration of endo-(1-4)-β-glucanase protected in a special environment in the immediate vicinity of the bacterial cell, or an endo-(1-4)-β-glucanase held in the correct configuration on the cellulose crystallite by the bacterium" may effect complete native cellulose solubilization.

The cellulolytic activities present in the culture supernatant of *A. cellulolyticus* were found to be greater than those obtained with commercial fungal preparations (25) but less than those from culture supernatants of highly cellulolytic mutants of *Trichoderma reesei*. Similarly, the crude extracellular cellulase of *C. thermocellum* strain LQRI solubilized microcrystalline cellulose at one-half the rate observed for the extracellular cellulase of *T. reesei* strain QM9414 (17). Strain selection methodologies similar to those employed in the production of hypercellulolytic *T. reesei* strains (14) offer enormous potential for the production of cellulases with high specific activity from anaerobic cellulolytic organisms. Enhanced cellulase synthesis and activity could also be accomplished by the application of genetic engineering techniques. This requires that genetic systems be developed for these anaerobes, and some progress is being made in this area. *C. thermocellum* genes coding for cellulose hydrolysis have been cloned and expressed in *Escherichia coli* (4). The sequence of a *C.thermocellum* cellulase gene has recently been determined (3).

The addition of β-glucosidase to cellulase preparations has been reported to have a stimulatory effect on the rate of cellulolysis (28). The extracellular cellulases from anaerobes do not exhibit β-glucosidase activity. The β-glucosidases of *C. thermocellum* (1), *B.succinogenes* (7), *R.lavefaciens* (24) *A.cellulolyticus* (12) and *R. albus* (19) are cell associated. The supplementation of cellulases derived from cellulolytic anaerobes with exogenous β-glucosidase may have potential in commercial saccharification processes.

CHEMICAL AND FUEL PRODUCTION BY CELLULOLYTIC ANAEROBES

Three systems for the biological conversion of cellulose into chemicals and fuels can be described:

<u>Indirect</u>. Saccharification by cellulase preparations. Fermentation of resultant released sugar eg. Ethanol production by *Saccharomyces cerevisiae*.

<u>Direct</u>. Saccharification and sugar fermentation by axenic cultures. e.g. Ethanol production by *C. thermocellum*.

<u>Coupled</u>. a) <u>Two-membered culture fermentation</u>. Saccharification and fermentation by a cellulolytic organism coupled to further transformations of resulting fermentation products and/or released sugar by non-cellulolytic organism. e.g. Methane production by *C. thermocellum* and *Methanobacterium thermoautotrophicum*.

b) <u>Multi-component fermentation</u>. Saccharification, fermentation and transformations of released sugars and fermentation products accomplished by a metabolic diverse range of organisms. e.g. Complete conversion of cellulose to methane by digesters.

Pure culture fermentations of cellulose by cellulolytic anaerobes result in a limited range of products.
Formate, acetate, butyrate, lactate, ethanol, succinate,
hydrogen and carbon dioxide have all been identified as
major fermentation products of axenic cultures of cellulolytic anaerobes (2,21,23,26,27,29). These compounds all
find use in various industrial processes (33). Ethanol,
for example, is important in the manufacture of laboratory
and industrial solvents, rubbing compounds, lotions,
colognes and, of increasing importance, octane booster in
gasoline. Anaerobic fermentations are characterized by a
high efficiency of conversion of substrates into products.
The transformation of cellulose carbon by cellulolytic
anaerobes into any particular fermentation product is
however limited. *A. cellulolyticus* and *C. thermocellum*
produce 0.78 mole (11) and 0.55 mole (29) of ethanol
respectively per mole of glucose equivalent fermented. In
contrast,the non-cellulolytic anaerobes *Thermoanaerobacter
ethanolicus* and *C. thermohydrosulfuricum* can produce up to
1.9 mole and 1.6 mole of ethanol respectively per mole of
sugar utilized (31). Direct fermentation for the production of ethanol is probably of limited significance.
Coupled fermentation systems, as discussed by Wiegel (31),
offer far greater potential for ethanol production from
cellulose. Soluble sugars produced during cellulose hydrolysis by the extracellular cellulase of the cellulolytic
anaerobe providing the carbon source for the ethanologenic
organism. A similar coupled fermentation system has been
suggested for the production of acetone and butanol from
cellulose (22).

The potential exists for the design of a range of
defined fermentation systems for the indirect or coupled

conversion of cellulose into chemicals and fuels of interest. The application of this technology is dependent on the availability of anaerobic microorganisms with desired metabolic characteristics, and on, a thorough understanding of their biochemistry.

CONCLUSIONS

Cellulose is the most important bio-polymer present in renewable biomass and therefore the most significant substrate for the production of chemicals and fuels by biological processes. Saccharification of cellulose by cellulases has many advantages over chemical hydrolysis but requires that the enzymes be cheaply produced. This may be obviated by coupled fermentation systems.

The economic feasibility of biological production of chemicals and fuels from renewable resources will be significantly improved by the conversion of both cellu- losic and non-cellulosic fractions. Starch, protein and hemicellulose are readily metabolized under anaerobic conditions whilst lignin is recalcitrant. The digesti- bility of cellulose is related to its degree of associa- tion with lignin. A delignification procedure, prior to fermentation, would greatly enhance the efficiency of conversion of cellulosic material into vendable products. The utilization of lignin-derived compounds as chemical feedstocks (8) would increase the cost-effectiveness of the overall biomass fermentation process. The future for the production of chemicals and fuels from renewable resources by biological means is promising. The next few decades will see whether this promise is fulfilled.

References

1 Ait, N., Creuzet, N. and Cattaneo, J. 1982.
   Properties of β-glucosidase from *Clostridium
   thermocellum*. J. Gen. Microbiol. 128: 569-577.

2 Bauchop, T. and Mountfort, D.O. 1981. Cellulose
   fermentation by a rumen anaerobic fungus in both the
   absence and presence of rumen methanogens. Appl.
   Environ. Microbiol. 42: 1103-1110.

3 Be'guin, P., Cornet, P. and Aubert, J-P. 1985.
   Sequence of a cellulase gene of the thermophilic
   bacterium *Clostridium thermocellum*.
   J. Bacteriol. 162: 102-105.

4 Cornet, P., Tronik, D., Millet, J. and Aubert, J-P.
   1983. Cloning and expression in *Escherichia coli* of
   Clostridium thermocellum genes coding for amino acid
   synthesis and cellulose hydrolysis.
   FEMS Microbiol. Letts. 16: 137-141.

5 Dunlap, C.E. and Chiang, L-C. 1980. Cellulose
   degradation-a common link. In: M.L. Shuler (ed.).
   Utilization and Recycle of Agricultural Wastes and
   Residues. CRC Press Inc. Boca Raton. p19.

6 Giallo, J., Gaudin, C. and Belaich, J-P. 1985.
   Metabolism and solubilization of cellulose by
   Clostridium cellulolyticus H10.
   Appl. Environ. Microbiol. 49: 1216-1221.

7 Groleau, D. and Forsberg. 1981. Cellulolytic
   activity of the rumen bacterium *Bacteroides
   succinogenes*. Can. J. Microbiol. 27: 517-530.

8 Hanselmann, K.W. 1982. Lignochemicals.
   Experientia. 35: 176-189.

9 Hobson, P.N., Bousfield, S. and Summers, R. 1981.
   Methane Production from Agricultural and Domestic
   Wastes. Applied Science Publishers. London.

10 Hungate, R.E. 1957. Microorganisms in the rumen of
    cattle fed a constant ration.
    Can. J. Microbiol. 3: 259-311.

11 Laube, M. and Martin, S.M. 1981. Conversion of
    cellulose to methane and carbon dioxide by triculture
    of *Acetivibrio cellulolyticus*, *Desulfovibrio* sp., and
    Methanosarcina barkeri.
    Appl. Environ. Microbiol. 42: 413-420.

12 MacKenzie, C.R. and Bilous, D. 1982. Location and
    kinetic properties of the cellulase system of
    Acetivibrio cellulolyticus.
    Can. J. Microbiol. 25: 1158-1164.

13 McCarty, P.L., Baugh, K., Bachmann, A., Owen, W. and
    Everhart, T. 1981. Autohydrolysis for increasing
    methane yields for lignocellulosic materials. In:
    D.L. Wise (ed.). Fuel Gas Developments. CRC Press
    Inc. Boca Raton. p49.

14   Montencourt, B.S. and Eveleigh, D.E.   1977.
      Preparation of mutants of *Trichoderma reesei* with
      enhanced cellulase production.
      Appl. Environ. Microbiol.   34: 777-782.

15   Mountfort, D.O. and Asher, R.A. 1985.   Production and
      regulation of cellulase by two strains of the rumen
      anaerobic fungus *Neocallimastix frontalis*.
      Appl. Environ. Microbiol. 49: 1314-1322.

16   Ng, A.S., Wong., D.Y., Stenstrom, M.K., Larson, L.
      and Mah, R.A. 1981. Bioconversion of classified
      municipal solid wastes: state-of-the-art review.
      In: D.L. Wise (ed.). Fuel Gas Developments. CRC Press
      Inc. Boca Raton. p73.

17   Ng, T.K. and Zeikus, J.G. 1981.   Comparision of
      extracellular cellulase activities of *Clostridium
      thermocellum* LQRI and *Trichoderma reesei* QM9414.
      Appl. Environ. Microbiol. 42: 231-240.

18   Ng, T.K., Weimer, P.J. and Zeikus, J.G.   1977.
      Cellulolytic and physiological properties of
      Clostridium thermocellum.
      Arch. Microbiol. 114: 1-7.

19   Ohmiya, K., Shirai, M., Kurachi, Y. and Shimizu, S.
      1985.   Isolation and properties of β-glucosidase
      from *Ruminococcus albus*.
      J. Bacteriol. 161: 432-434.

20   Orpin, C.G. and Letcher, A.J. 1979.   Utilization of
      cellulose, starch, xylan and other hemicelluloses for
      growth by the rumen phycomycete *Neocallimastix
      frontalis*.   Curr. Microbiol. 3: 121-124.

21   Patel, G.B., Khan, A.W., Agnew, B.J. and Colvin, J.R.
      1980.   Isolation and characterization of an anaerobic
      cellulolytic microorganism, *Acetivibrio
      cellulolyticus* gen. nov., sp. nov.
      Int. J. Syst. Bacteriol. 30: 179-185.

22   Petitdemange, E., Fond, O., Caillet, F.,
      Petitdemange, H. and Gay, R.   1983.   A novel one-
      step process for cellulose fermentation using
      mesophilic cellulolytic and glycolytic clostridia.
      Biotechnol. Letts. 5: 119-124.

23   Petitdemange, E., Caillet, F., Giallo, J. and Gaudin.
      C. 1984.   *Clostridium cellulolyticum* sp. nov., a
      cellulolytic, mesophilic species from decayed grass.
      Int. J. Syst.Bacteriol. 34: 155-159

24   Pettipher, G.L. and Latham, M.J.   1979.
      Characteristics of enzymes produced by *Ruminococcus
      flavefaciens* which degrade plant cell walls.
      J. Gen. Microbiol. 110: 21-27.

25   Saddler, J.N. and Khan, A.W. 1980.   Cellulase
      production by *Acetivibrio cellulolyticus*.
      Can. J. Microbiol. 26: 760-765.

26   Sleat, R. and Mah. R.A.   1988.   *Clostridium populeti*
      sp. nov., a cellulolytic species from a woody-biomass
      digester.   Int. J. Syst. Bacteriol.   35: 160-163.

27   Sleat, R., Mah, R.A. and Robinson, R.   1984.
      Isolation and characterization of an anaerobic,
      cellulolytic bacterium, *Clostridium cellulovorans* sp.
      nov.   Appl. Environ. Microbiol. 48: 88-93.

28   Sternberg, D., Vivayakumar, P. and Reese, E.   1976.
       β-glucosidase microbial production and effect on
      enzymatic hydrolysis of cellulose.
      Can. J. Microbiol. 23: 139-147.

29   Weimer, P.J. and Zeikus, J.G.   1977.   Fermentation of
      cellulose and cellobiose by *Clostridium thermocellum*
      in the absence and presence of *Methanobacterium*
      thermoautotrophicum.   Appl. Environ. Microbiol. 33: 289-297.

30   West, C.E., Ashare, E. and Langton, E.H. 1981.
      Feasibility study for anaerobic digestion of
      agricultural crop residues for fuel gas. In: D.L.
      Wise (ed.). Fuel Gas Developments. CRC Press Inc.
      p201.

31   Wiegel, J. 1982.   Ethanol from cellulose.
      Experientia. 38: 151-156.

32   Wood, T.M. and Wilson,C.A.   1984.   Some properties
      of the endo-(1-4)- β -D-glucanase synthesized by
      the anaerobic cellulolytic rumen bacterium
      Ruminococcus albus.   Can. J. Microbiol. 80: 816-821.

33   Zeikus, J.G. 1980.   Chemical and fuel production by
      anaerobic bacteria. Ann. Rev. Microbiol. 84: 423-464.

SECTION 5. ANAEROBES AND GENITAL TRACT INFECTIONS.

Chairman of session : Professor C.S.F. Easman

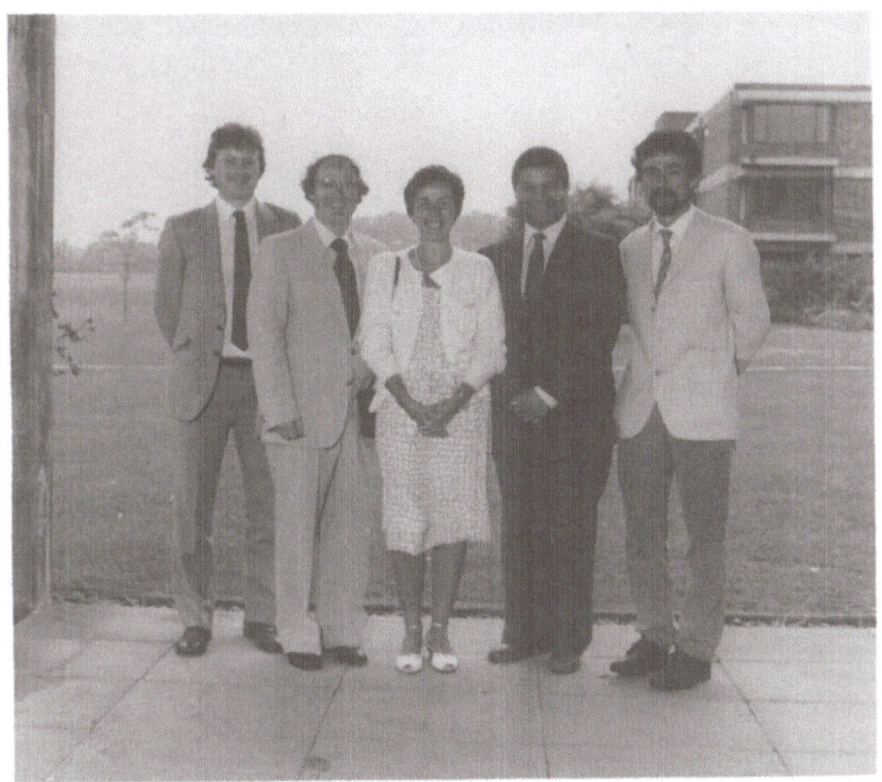

From left to right :

T. Winstanley, B.I. Duerden, Ada Vetere, C.S.F. Easman and M. Wilkes

CHAPTER   17

THE ANAEROBIC BACTERIAL FLORA OF THE VAGINA IN HEALTH AND DISEASE.

Mark Wilks and Soad Tabaqchali

Department of Medical Microbiology, St. Bartholomews Hospital
Medical College, West Smithfield, London, EC1A 7BE, UK.

Contents

Abstract

Introduction

Patients and methods

    Patients

    Sampling

    Processing of specimens

    Enumeration and identification of organisms

Results

    Vaginal flora in health.

    Vaginal flora in genital disease.

Discussion

References

ABSTRACT

A quantitative sampling method was used to analyse the vaginal flora from healthy women and women with a variety of genital diseases.

Single samples were taken from 30 asymptomatic women, the mean total bacterial count was 8.4 $\log_{10}$ cfu/g consisting of 8.2 $\log_{10}$ cfu/g anaerobes and 7.4 $\log_{10}$ cfu/g aerobes. The vaginal flora was composed predominantly of aerobic and anaerobic lactobacilli, coryneforms, *Staphylococcus epidermidis*, *Bacteroides* spp., *Bifidobacteria*, and anaerobic Gram-positive cocci. In multiple samples taken throughout the menstrual cycle from ten of these asymptomatic women the mean number of species decreased significantly from a mean of 5.4 at the beginning of the cycle to 3.6 at the end, but the bacterial counts did not change.

The bacterial flora of 82 women with a variety of different genital diseases was essentially similar with anaerobes outnumbering aerobes by about one log unit except in women with gonorrhoea or who were contacts of men with non-specific urethritis (NSU). However, a combination of *Gardnerella vaginalis* and anaerobic Gram-positive cocci was found in seven out of 14 patients with non specific vaginitis (NSV) and in five out of 16 NSU contact patients but only occasionally in other genital diseases and in asymptomatic women. There were no particular changes in the vaginal flora associated with the presence of known pathogens such as *Neisseria gonorrhoeae*, *Trichomonas vaginalis* and *Candida albicans*. Lactobacilli did not confer any protective effect by excluding the presence of other possible pathogens such as *G. vaginalis* or anaerobes.

INTRODUCTION

Although the presence of anaerobic bacteria in the female genital tract has been known since the 1920's, most studies have used methods which are more suitable for the isolation of the aerobic components of the vaginal flora. The purpose of this paper is to describe some of the work that has been done over the last few years on the bacterial vaginal flora using quantitative sampling methods and techniques suitable for the isolation of anaerobes over in the Departments of Medical Microbiology and Genital Medicine (DGM) at St. Bartholomew's Hospital.

PATIENTS AND METHODS.

Patients. Patients were grouped according to their disease syndromes and the pathogens isolated, i.e. gono-coccal disease (GC), *Trichomonas vaginalis* (TV), candida, non-specific vaginitis (NSV), non-specific genital infection (NSGI), non-specific urethritis contacts (NSUC) and a control group. Women who had taken anti-microbials in the preceeding month were excluded. Patient's age, stage of menstrual cycle, contraceptive practice and parity were also recorded. Patients from whom two or more pathogens were isolated e.g. *N.gonorrhoeae* and *T.vaginalis* were omitted from this report. Because of confusion which has arisen from inadequate definition of patient groups in the past, some of the definitions used in this study are given at length. NSV was defined as the presence of an abnormal amount of vaginal discharge, without specifying colour, with or without inflammation of the vaginal mucosa (as judged by one clinician), in the absence of other

pathogens and of any contact with any known sexually
transmitted disease. In addition these patients did not
have a gross excess of leukocytes in the Gram-stained
cervical smear, nor did they have inflammatory changes
affecting the epithelial cells on the Papanicolau-stained
cervical smears. NSGI was defined as the presence of a
gross excess of leukocytes, inflammatory changes affecting
epithelial cells, the absence of GC, TV or candida and the
absence of contact with any known sexually transmitted
disease.

The control group consisted of women attending a nearby
family planning clinic for contraceptive advice who agreed
to participate in the study and asymptomatic healthy
volunteers who attended the DGM at this hospital in
response to a request for volunteers. In addition, single
samples were also taken from three women attending the DGM
who had no excess of vaginal discharge, no GC, TV or
candida, none of the inflammatory changes noted in
patients with NSGI and no known contact with any sexually
transmitted disease. Multiple samples were taken from ten
of the volunteers. These women were chosen because they
had a regular menstrual cycle of about 28 days and were
not taking oral contraceptives. The first sample was
taken around the beginning of the cycle when menstruation
had ceased or virtually ceased. The remaining three
samples were taken at weekly intervals after that.

Sampling. After evaluating several existing quantitative
methods and encountering difficulties with all of them, we
developed our own method which has been described in
detail elsewhere (5). Briefly, samples were collected
from the posterior vaginal fornix using a standard bacteriological loop. They were then placed in pre-weighed

tubes of modified Cary-Blair medium which had been prepared in the anaerobic chamber, and the tube and contents re-weighed.

Processing of specimens. The tube was passed into the anaerobic chamber, sterile glass beads added and the specimen homogenised on a rotamixer. The specimens were then diluted in VPI dilution blanks (2) and 100 microlitre aliquots spread onto the surface of Brucella blood agar, neomycin blood agar, kanamycin-vancomycin blood agar and Rogosa agar which had been prepared in the anaerobic chamber. The tubes were removed from the chamber and 100 microlitre samples spread onto the surface of Blood, MacConkey, modified Thayer-Martin, and colistin-nalidixic acid human blood agar for aerobic incubation.

Enumeration and identification of organisms. Anaerobic plates were incubated for up to seven days at 35°C in the chamber. Aerobic plates were incubated for two or three days at 35°C in an atmosphere of air + CO_2 (5%). After incubation different colony types were enumerated and subcultured for identification by previously described methods (6). Bacterial counts were expressed as the logarithm of the number of colony-forming units per gram (log_{10} cfu/g).

RESULTS

Vaginal flora in health. a. Single samples. The quantitative vaginal flora of the 30 women in the control group is summarised in Table 1. The mean total bacterial count was 8.4 log_{10} cfu/g, anaerobes outnumbering aerobes by almost one log unit. Lactobacilli were the most common isolates, mainly aerobic strains, but a substantial number of anaerobic strains were also isolated. *Bacteroides* of

Table 1. Quantitative vaginal flora of 30 healthy women.

	Mean count (log₁₀ cfu/g)	Number(%) of samples positive
Total bacteria	8.4	30 (100)
Anaerobes	8.2	28 (93)
Lactobacilli	7.3	19 (63)
B. bivius/disiens	7.4	15 (50)
Anaerobic gpc	6.4	8 (27)
Bifidobacteria	7.5	7 (23)
Aerobes	7.4	30 (100)
Lactobacilli	7.4	26 (87)
S.epidermidis	7.4	19 (63)
Coryneforms	6.9	15 (50)
G.vaginalis	6.2	4 (13)

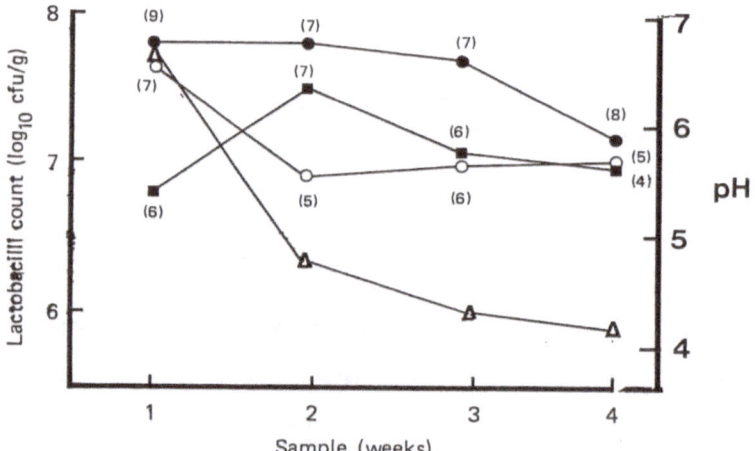

Figure 1. Incidence and concentration of lactobacilli during the menstrual cycle.
● Total lactobacilli   ○ Anaerobic strains
■ Aerobic strains   △ pH
( ) Number of specimens positive

the *B. bivius/disiens* group were isolated from half of the patients. Other species of *Bacteroides* were not as common. *G. vaginalis* was only isolated from four of the 30 samples (13%).

b. <u>Multiple samples</u>. There were no great differences between the total counts from week to week (Figure 1), although the mean number of species isolated per specimen declined significantly during the cycle from a mean of 5.8 in week one to 4.8 in week two, 4.6 in week three and 3.6 in week four. This decline was not due to any one organism or group of organisms in particular. The incidence and concentration of aerobic and anaerobic strains of lactobacilli for each of the weeks of the cycle and the mean vaginal pH are shown in Figure 2. It can be seen that there is a rapid decrease in vaginal pH from week one to week two.

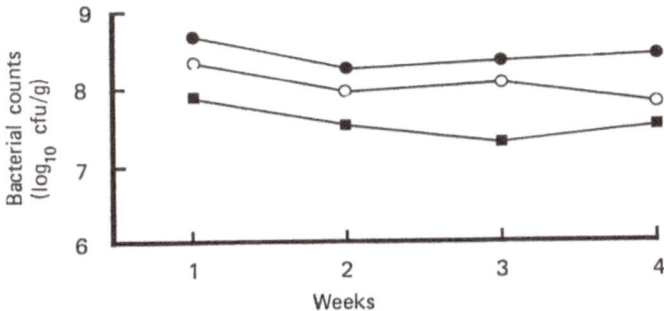

Figure 2. Bacterial counts during the menstrual cycle of ten healthy women. ● Total ■ Aerobes ○ Anaerobes.

Vaginal flora in genital diseases. The results of single
samples from women with a range of the different genital
diseases are summarised in Table 2. The control group is
shown again for comparison. All the patients had aerobes
and nearly all had anaerobes. The anaerobes outnumbered
aerobes typically by about one log unit except in the GC
and NSUC groups where the differences are not so great.
G. vaginalis was isolated from eight out of the 14
patients with NSV and in six of 16 NSUC patients but was
much less common in the other conditions. The presence of
G.vaginalis in these two groups appeared to correlate with
a high incidence and concentration of anaerobic Gram-
positive cocci. The occurrence of bacteroides did not

Table 2. Quantitative vaginal bacterial flora in genital disease.

	GC (11)*	TV (17)	Candida (17)	NSV (14)	NSUC (16)	NSGI (7)	Control group (30)
Total bacteria	8.2 (11)	8.7 (17)	7.8 (17)	8.3 (14)	8.2 (16)	8.3 (7)	8.4 (30)
Total aerobes	7.7 (11)	7.3 (17)	7.0 (17)	7.2 (17)	7.3 (16)	7.0 (7)	7.4 (30)
Total anaerobes	8.0 (11)	8.7 (17)	7.8 (17)	8.3 (13)	7.6 (16)	8.3 (6)	8.2 (28)
G. vaginalis	7.3 (2)	5.7 (2)	7.8 (1)	7.0 (8)	7.4 (6)	6.8 (1)	6.2 (4)
Anaerobic Gram-positive cocci	7.9 (5)	8.7 (9)	6.8 (6)	7.7 (10)	7.2 (10)	7.7 (5)	6.4 (15)
Bacteroides spp	6.5 (2)	7.7 (5)	4.8 (3)	7.1 (4)	5.9 (7)	7.7 (4)	7.4 (15)

* = number of subjects in group

correlate with any particular genital disease such as TV
as has been found by some workers (1), nor was it

associated with a particular organism such as *G. vaginalis*
as reported by Spiegel and co-workers (4).

DISCUSSION.

The vaginal flora in healthy women has traditionally
been regarded as being aerobic and consisting largely of
lactobacilli, which are thought to produce lactic acid by
splitting glycogen deposited in the vaginal epithelium by
the action of oestrogen. The acidity produced is considered
to be important in restricting the growth of other organisms.
In this study, lactobacilli were found to be the most
common organisms, however there was also a well developed
anaerobic flora in healthy women and women with a range of
genital diseases. The pathogenic significance of the
anaerobic flora is not certain. Some workers have suggested
that anaerobes have a protective role, preventing the
growth of potential pathogens as in the gastro-intestinal
tract (3). Others have suggested that the presence of
anaerobes themselves is of pathogenic significance, either
causing disease or associated with it. We found a combination of *G. vaginalis* and anaerobic Gram-positive cocci
in seven out of 14 patients with NSV and in five out 16
NSUC patients. This combination was rarely found in the
other groups or in the control group. However anaerobic
Gram-positive cocci in the absence of *G. vaginalis* was a
common finding in all the patient groups including the
control group. From our work we conclude that the mere
presence of anaerobes in the vagina should not be regarded
as being of pathogenic significance.

ACKNOWLEDGEMENTS

We thank Dr R.N. Thin, formerly Consultant in Charge, Department of Genital Medicine, St. Bartholomews Hospital for clinical
assessment of the patients. This study was supported by the Joint
Research Board of St Bartholomews Hospital.

References

1   Goldacre, M.J. Watt, B., Loudon, N., Milne, L.J.R.,
    Loudon, J.D.O. and Vessey, M.P.   1979. Vaginal
    microbial flora in normal young women.
    Br. med. J. 1: 1450-1453.

2   Holdeman, L.V., Cato, E.P., and Moore, W.E.C. 1977.
    Anaerobe Laboratory Manual, 4th ed. Virginia
    Polytechnic Institute and State University Blacksburg.

3   Larsen, B. and Galask, R.P. 1982. Vaginal microbial
    flora: composition and influence of host physiology.
    Ann. Intern. Med. 96: 926-930.

4   Spiegel, C.A., Amsel, R., Eschenbach, D, Schoenknecht,
    F. and Holmes, K.K. 1980. Anaerobic bacteria in non-
    specific vaginitis. N. Eng. J. Med. 303: 601-607.

5   Wilks, M., Thin, R.N., and Tabaqchali, S. 1982.
    Quantitative methods for studies on the vaginal flora.
    J. Med. Microbiol. 15: 141-147.

6   Wilks, M., Thin, R.N., and Tabaqchali, S. 1984.
    Quantitative bacteriology of the vaginal flora in
    genital disease.   J. Med. Microbiol. 18: 217-231.

CHAPTER 18

MOBILUNCUS AND BACTERIAL VAGINOSIS.

Ada Vetere*, S. P. Borriello[1] and D. Taylor-Robinson,

[1] Divisions of Sexually Transmitted Diseases and Communicable
Diseases, Clinical Research Centre, Watford Road, Harrow, Middlesex,
HA1 3UJ, UK.

*Present Address Clinica Medica III, Policlinico Umberto I,
Universita di Roma, Viale dell'Universita 37, 00185 Rome, Italy.

Contents

Abstract

Introduction

Materials and Methods

Results

Conclusion

References

206

ABSTRACT

Anaerobic, curved, motile, Gram-negative organism, belonging to a "new" genus have been isolated recently from up to 50% of women with bacterial vaginosis, suggesting that they might play an important role in the pathogenesis of the syndrome. The organisms have been given the genus name *Mobiluncus* and two species are recognised at present: *Mobiluncus curtisii* and *M.mulieris*.

We studied 33 strains of *Mobiluncus* spp. isolated from the urogenital tract. We found that the best growth occurred after five days of anaerobic incubation at 37°C on Columbia blood agar, while the best selective medium appeared to be CNA agar supplemented with 50mcg/ml of aztreonam.

Five of the 24 isolates identified as *M. curtisii* and four of the nine isolates identified as *M. mulieris* produced atypical biochemical reactions in comparison with the results reported by the majority of other workers. Our results support the hypothesis that the genus *Mobiluncus* may consist of more than two species and also confirm the fastidiousness of these organisms.

Further studies will be needed to assess the effectiveness of our selective medium, the use of which could help to clarify the role of the organisms in bacterial vaginosis, and establish whether they are sexually transmitted.

INTRODUCTION

The new genus *Mobiluncus* comprises anaerobic, curved, motile, Gram-variable, non-spore-forming rods which are of particular interest because they have been isolated from up to 50% of patients with bacterial vaginosis.

This syndrome consists of at least three of the following features in women with vaginal complaints: a homogeneous and thin vaginal discharge, a vaginal pH value greater than 4.5, a discharge with a typical "fishy" odour, and a smear of the discharge in which there are bacteria-coated cells ("clue cells").

The presence of motile curved rods in vaginal smears was first reported in 1895 by Kronig, but it was not until 1980 that Durieux and Dublanchet (3) isolated and cultured these types of organisms from a significant number of patients with vaginosis. Since then almost all those who have studied this syndrome have reported the presence of anaerobic curved rods with isolation rates of 14% to 50% in women with disease and about 5% in healthy women (3,8,10,11). Furthermore, the presence of these bacteria correlates with features of an altered vaginal flora, such as a diminished number of lactobacilli and an increased number of other anaerobes, such as *Bacteroides* and *Peptococci* (10,11). It is also of interest to note that in the most recent studies, *Mobiluncus* organisms were found frequently in association with *Gardnerella vaginalis* (7).

The current opinion is that the genus *Mobiluncus* comprises two distinct species, (12) each identified by their cellular morphology, Gram-staining, biochemical activity and metronidazole susceptibility: they are *M.curtisii* (short form) and *M. mulieris* (long form).

SDS-PAGE, DNA-DNA hybridization and serological techniques also differentiate *Mobiluncus* into two definite species, but so far there is no absolutely unanimous consensus on the differentiative criteria for the two forms.

Mobiluncus organisms are very fastidious on primary isolation, forming only very small colonies (1-2 microns in diameter) after three to four days of anaerobic incubation. In the laboratory processing of clinical specimens containing an abundant and complex endogenous flora, such as vaginal discharges, it is very difficult and sometimes impossible to recognize colonies of *Mobiluncus*. Furthermore, the isolation of these organisms in pure culture is frequently lengthy (3) sometimes taking several weeks (15).

In the attempt to clarify the problem of differentiating between the two forms, to find their best growth conditions, and to discover an effective selective medium to facilitate their isolation, we studied 33 strains of *Mobiluncus* spp.

MATERIALS AND METHODS

All the strains received were isolated from patients with bacterial vaginosis, except one which was isolated from the seminal fluid of an infertile man.

The growth of all strains was tested in a range of both solid and liquid media. In addition. arginine, sodium hippurate, formate-fumarate, bovine serum and Campylobacter growth supplement-FBP were added individually to Brain heart infusion broth to screen for potential growth enhancement activity. Growth at different temperatures, in different atmospheres, and at different pH values was examined also.

The susceptibility of the strains to 30 antimicrobials was tested by the disc-diffusion technique.

A range of biochemical reactions was assayed by use of the new API AN3 test strip which contains 14 carbohydrates, and the API 20 kit for an additional eight sugars. Thirty-seven enzyme activities were tested with the API ZYM kit and with the new API AN1, AN2 and AN3 test strips.

RESULTS

The optimum growth conditions were provided by Columbia blood agar in an anaerobic atmosphere at 37°C or 33°C: no strain grew at 42°C or under aerobic incubation. Growth of all strains occurred also after five days incubation in 5% O_2 in nitrogen at 37°C. There was no growth at pH values lower than 6.0, the optimum occurring at pH values from 6.5 to 8.0.

These results might explain the reported low rate of isolation of these organisms from the vagina of healthy women (10,11,8), as the normal vaginal environment never has a pH value higher than 4.5; it seems that the increasing vaginal pH in bacterial vaginosis (mainly due to smaller number of lactobacilli) may facilitate growth of *Mobiluncus* organisms.

The major differentiative criteria for *Mobiluncus* spp. are shown in table 1. According to the majority of

Table 1. Distinction between *M. curtissi* and *M. mulieris.*

Reactions	*M. curtisii*	*M. mulieris*
β – galactosidase	+	−
Hippurate hydrolysis	+	−
Arginine hydrolysis	+	−
Leucine aminopeptidase	−	+
Metronidazole (MICs)	16–1000 mcg/ml (5mcg discs R)	0.5–4 mcg/ml (5mcg discs S)

published work, the short forms (*M.curtisii*) show positive reactions for arginine and hippurate hydrolysis and for β -galactosidase, and are resistant to metronidazole, while the long forms (*M. mulieris*) are negative in all these tests and sensitive to metronidazole. We did not find, however, such a clear cut distinction with all our strains. Of the 33 strains examined, 19 had typical reactions of *M. curtisii* and five of *M.mulieris*. However, five short forms had atypical reactions for *M. curtisii*; two were negative for β -galactosidase, two for hippurate hydrolysis and one for arginine hydrolysis. In addition, four long forms had atypical reactions for *M. mulieris* in that three of them were resistant to metronidazole: one of these was positive for β -galactosidase activity and arginine hydrolysis: one was biochemically identical to a typical *M.curtisii* and another was biochemically identical to a typical *M. mulieris*. The only atypical *M. mulieris* sensitive to metronidazole was positive in the hippurate hydrolysis test. Because of the peculiarity of these findings, we repeated all tests on at least three different occasions, but always obtained the same results.

The possibility that *Mobiluncus* spp. could be divided into more than two groups has been raised recently by several workers (5), and DNA-DNA hybridization studies have supported a sub-speciation of the short forms, the long forms seeming to be a more heterogeneous group than the short forms (2). We believe that a categorical division of these organisms into two groups is not satisfactory and that the possibility of atypical results, even for metronidazole susceptibility, should always be considered.

The fermentation pattern shows that typical strains of

M. curtisii are almost inert, fermenting only ribose and xylose, while typical strains of *M. mulieris* ferment a range of carbohydrates. The atypical short and long forms have a fermentation pattern similar to that of the typical long forms (*M. mulieris*) differing only for trehalose fermentation. α -methyl-D-glucoside fermentation could be a useful test to distinguish both typical and atypical strains of *M. curtisii*, all of which are negative, from the typical and atypical strains of *M. mulieris*, which generally are positive.

A biochemical reaction profile obtained by analysis for preformed enzymes showed that all strains of *Mobiluncus* were positive for leucine aminopeptidase the amino acid arylamidases and tetrathionate reductase, but negative for α -D-fucosidase, trypsin, phospho-β -galactosidase and naphthol-ASBi-phosphate. In general, typical strains of *M. curtisii* were less reactive than those of *M. mulieris*.

The antibiotic susceptibility of these strains is atypical for Gram-negative organisms: in fact, they are sensitive to bacitracin and vancomycin, as are the majority of Gram-positive anaerobes, while they are resistant to colistin sulphate and aztreonam. To date only some *Bacteroides* organisms of the melaninogenicus group and a few other *Bacteroides* spp have been reported to have antibiotic susceptibilities similar to these (13). On the other hand, electron-microscopy of their cell-wall structure shows that they do not have any outer membrane (in contrast to Gram-negative bacteria) and that they differ from typical Gram-positive organisms in having some electron-dense zone within the wall structure.

It seems likely that *Mobiluncus* spp. are Gram-positive

organisms that can be easily de-stained, in the same way as butyrivibrio and some coryneforms.

It is of particular interest that all the *Mobiluncus* strains were resistant to high concentrations of aztreonam (up to 50mcg/ml), a new cephalosporin active mainly against Gram-negative aerobes. Encouraged by this result, we prepared a selective medium by incorporating 50mcg/ml of aztreonam in CNA agar base. This medium is being evaluated.

CONCLUSION

In conclusion. the taxonomy of the genus *Mobiluncus* is still unclear and further studies will be needed to elucidate this problem. Furthermore, these organisms are very fastidious, and the development of an effective selective medium will be helpful in clarifying whether they have a pathogenic role in bacterial vaginosis and in establishing whether they are sexually transmitted.

References

1   Baron, E.J., Wexler, H.M. and Finegold, S. M.   1984.
     Biochemical and polyacrylamide gel electrophoretic
     analysis of vaginosis-associated anaerobic curved
     rods.   In: P-A. Mårdh and D. Taylor-Robinson (eds.).
     Bacterial Vaginosis.   Almqvist and Wiskell
     International.   Stockholm.   p. 65.

2   Christiansen, G., Hansen, E., Holst, E., Christiansen,
     C. and Mårdh, P.-A. 1984.   Genetic relationships of
     short and long anaerobic curved rods isolated from the
     vagina.   In: P-A. Mårdh and D. Taylor-Robinson
     (eds.).   Bacterial Vaginosis.   Aimqvist and Wiskell
     International.   Stockholm.   p. 75.

3   Durieux, R. and Dublanchet, A. 1980.   Les vibrions
     anaerobies des leucorrhees I: Technique de isolament
     et sensibilite aux antibiotiques.
     Med. Mal. Inf. 10: 109-

4   Fox, A. and Phillips. I.   1984.   Two curved rods in
     non-specific vaginosis. In: P-A. Mårdh and D. Taylor-
     Robinson (eds.) Bacterial Vaginosis. Almqvist and
     Wiskell international.   Stockholm.   p. 93.

5   Holst, E., Skarin. A. and Mårdh, P-A.   1982.
     Characteristics of anaerobic comma-shaped bacteria
     recovered from the female genital tract.
     Eur. J. Clin. Microbiol. 1: 310-16.

6   Moi, H. and Dannielson, D. 1984.   Studies on rabbit
     hyperimmune, patient and blood donor serum with regard
     to bactericidal activity and serum antibodies against
     anaerobic curved rods from patients with bacterial
     vaginosis.   in: P-A. Mårdh and D. Taylor-Robinson
     (eds.) Bacterial Vaginosis.   Aimqvist and Wiskell
     International.   Stockholm.   p. 89.

7   Pattman, R.S.   1984.   The significance of finding
     curved rods in the vaginal secretions of women
     attending a genito-urinary medical clinic.   In: P-A.
     Mårdh and D. Taylor-Robinson (eds.) Bacterial
     Vaginosis.   Aimqvist and Wiskell International.
     Stockholm.   p. 143.

8   Skarin, A. and Mårdh, P-A.   1982.   Comma-shaped
     bacteria associated with vaginitis.   Lancet.   1: 342.

9   Skarin, A., Larsson, L., Hoist, E.A. and Mardh, P.-A.
     1984.   Gas chromatographic analysis of cellular fatty
     acids in anaerobic curved bacteria isolated from
     vagina.   In: P-A. Mårdh and D. Taylor-Robinson (eds.).
     Bacterial Vaginosis.   Aimqvist and Wiskell
     International.   Stockholm.   p. 71.

10   Spiegel, C.A., Amsel, R., Eschenbach, D.,
     Schoenknecht, F. and Holmes. K.K. 1980.   Anaerobic
     bacteria in non-specific vaginosis.
     New Engl. J. Med. 303: 601-7.

11   Spiegel, C.A., Eschenbach, D., Amsel, R. and Holmes.
     K.K. 1983. Curved anaerobic bacteria in bacterial
     vaginosis and their response to antimicrobial therapy.
     J. Inf. Dis. 148: 81 7-22.

12   Spiegel, C.A. and Roberts, M. 1984. *Mobiluncus* gen.
     nov., *Mobiluncus curtisii* subsp, *curtisii* sp. nov.,
     Mobiluncus curtisii subsp. *holmesii* subsp. nov. and
     Mobiluncus mulieris sp. nov. curved rods from the
     human vagina. Int. J. Syst. Bacteriol. 34: 177-184.

13   Sutter, V.L., Citron, D.M. and Finegold, S.M. In:
     Wadsworth Anaerobic Bacteriology Manual. 3rd ed.
     Mosby Company. London.

14   Taylor, A.J. and Owen, R.J. 1984. Morphological and
     chemical characteristics of anaerobic comma-shaped
     rods from female genital tract. In: P-A. Mårdh and
     D. Taylor-Robinson (eds.). Bacterial Vaginosis.
     Almqvist and Wiskell International. Stockholm. p. 97.

15   Thomason, S.L., Schreckenberger, P.C.. Spellacy, W.N.
     Riff, L.S. and Le-Beau, L. J. 1984. Clinical and
     microbiological characterization of patients with non-
     specific vaginosis associated with motile, curved
     anaerobic rods. J. Inf. Dis. 149: 801-9.

CHAPTER 19

DIFFERENTIATION OF *MOBILUNCUS* SPECIES BY PYROLYSIS GAS-LIQUID CHROMATOGRAPHY

T.G. Winstanley, J.M. Hindmarch and J.T. Magee*

Department of Bacteriology, Royal Hallamshire Hospital, Sheffield, S10 2JF, UK.

* Department of Bacteriology, Children's Hospital, Western Bank, Sheffield, S10 2TH, UK.

Contents

Abstract

Introduction

Materials and Methods

    Strains

    Biochemical and morphological characterisation

    PGLC equipment

    Pyrolysis and GLC techniques

    Numerical analysis of data and identification program

Results

    Biochemistry and morphology

    Pyrolysis

Discussion

References

ABSTRACT

Vaginal anaerobic curved rods isolated from cases of bacterial vaginosis were characterised by morphology, biochemical tests and pyrolysis gas-liquid chromatography (PGLC). Classification of the strains based upon each of the above criteria independently showed division into two similar groups. Group I organisms were short, Gram-variable, comma-shaped rods, ONPG positive and able to hydrolyse arginine and hippurate. Group II organisms were long, Gram-negative, curved rods, ONPG negative and unable to hydrolyse arginine or hippurate. Each group produced a distinct PGLC pattern. These groups corresponded to the valid descriptions of *Mobiluncus curtisii* and *M.mulieris*. PGLC patterns of all other genera examined were not similar to those obtained for either group of anaerobic curved rods. The role of *Mobiluncus* species in disease processes remains obscure: characterisation studies such as this may lead to a better understanding of their significance in human infection.

INTRODUCTION

In 1895, Kronig observed comma-shaped bacteria in the vaginal flora (11). Curtis, in 1913, was the first to isolate motile curved anaerobic bacteria in pure culture (6). Two species of anaerobic curved rods can be distinguished on the basis of morphological, cultural and biochemical differences and these appear unrelated to previously described genera (8,18,24,25). DNA hybridisation

studies also indicate that the group can be divided into
two distinct species, with intra-species homologies of
>75% and inter-species homologies ranging from nine to 25%
(5). Sodium dodecyl sulphate-polyacrylamide gel electrophoresis (SDS-PAGE) peptide patterns of whole-cell extracts
are species specific and indicate a high intra-species
similarity (1). Strains from the same species are strongly
reactive with homologous antisera, but generally are weakly
reactive with antisera to the heterologous species (16).
These organisms have been classified in the genus Mobiluncus.
Two species have been proposed, *M. curtisii* (with subspecies
curtisii and *holmesii*) and *M. mulieris* (24). *Mobiluncus*
spp. are frequently isolated from cases of bacterial
vaginosis, although their role in the disease process, if
any, remains to be elucidated (3,8,20,23,25). The organisms
have also been isolated from extra-genital sites such as
breast abscesses and infected umbilical and mastectomy
wounds (9,26).

In pyrolysis, thermolytic cleavage of chemical bonds
in a specimen heated in an inert atmosphere yields a
mixture of low molecular weight products whose quantitative
and qualitative composition reflects the composition of
the specimen (7). In Curie-point pyrolysis, the heat is
produced by magnetic induction in a ferromagnetic carrier
coated with the specimen (4). The volatile products of
pyrolysis may be separated and quantitated by gas-liquid
chromatography (PGLC) or by mass spectrometry (PMS); the
use of these techniques in the characterisation of microorganisms has been reviewed by Gutteridge and Norris (10).
The application of PGLC to the characterisation of
Mobiluncus is presented here.

MATERIALS AND METHODS

<u>Strains</u>.   Anaerobic   curved rods were obtained from   the
collections   of Professor I.Phillips,   Dr M.Sprott and   Dr
A.Skarin.   The remaining 44 strains were isolated on non-
selective media,   from clinical specimens processed in the
routine   bacteriology laboratory at The Royal   Hallamshire
Hospital.   All organisms were isolated from patients with
bacterial   vaginosis   as defined by Blackwell   and   Barlow
(2).   Well-characterised   clinical strains representative
of other genera were also studied.

<u>Biochemical   and morphological characterisation</u>.   Unclass-
ified   anaerobic   curved rods (50) were   characterised   by
colony   morphology on Columbia agar (LabM) with   5%   horse
blood   (CBA) and by Gram stain.   All isolates were motile
by   the   hanging   drop   method.   Biochemical   tests   were
performed using methods outlined by Sprott and   co-workers
(25)   and   Levett (12).   Organisms were classified   using
cluster analysis (Jaccard coefficient,   UPGMA heirarchical
fusion) of morphological and biochemical data.

<u>PGLC   equipment</u>.   A Pye-Unicam series   PU4500   gas-liquid
chromatograph (Pye-Unicam,   York Street,   Cambridge,   CB1
2PX)   with   dual   flame   ionisation   detectors,   gas   flow
control unit, temperature programming unit, and a Phillips
8251 chart recorder,   was in routine use for the identification of anaerobes.   To this were added (i) a Pye-Unicam
Curie   point   pyrolyser,   (ii) an   eight-bit   analogue   to
digital converter(ADC), (iii) a Commodore 64 microcomputer
(Commodore   Systems,   675 Ajax   Avenue,   Trading   Estate,
Slough, Bucks) and (iv) a Commodore 1525 dot-matrix printer.
The ADC transmitted a 0-255 digital output to the computer,
corresponding to a zero to twice full scale deflection   of
the   chart recorder pen.   The computer was programmed   to

measure the retention times and heights of the peaks and
to print these after each analysis.

Pyrolysis and GLC technique. Test strains were grown
anaerobically for 72hr at 37°C on CBA. Colonies were
picked from the surface of the agar directly onto a flamed
pyrolysis wire (Curie point 610°C, Pye-Unicam). The wire,
with its attached septum, was inserted into the chromatograph. During this procedure, the column injection port
was left open with nitrogen carrier gas flowing to prevent
entry of air into the column. A period of 3 min was
allowed for re-stabilisation of the carrier gas flow rate
and drying of the specimen. Then, an 8 second period of
pyrolysis, the chromatograph temperature program and the
computer peak recording routine were started simultaneously.
The chromatography conditions were: injection oven temperature 190°C, detector oven temperature 230°C and column
oven temperature 80°C for 2min followed by a programmed
increase of 12°C/min to a final temperature of 200°C which
was held for 6min. Detector gas flow rates were, hydrogen
25ml/min and air 250ml/min. The pyrolysis column flow
rate was 25ml/min. Fine daily adjustments of the carrier
gas flow-rates were made with a bubble flowmeter. The
balance column flow-rate was adjusted to give a small
positive baseline shift over the temperature program in a
blank run. The computer recorded this baseline shift and
subtracted an appropriate correction from each peak height
recorded in subsequent pyrograms during that day. The
baseline shift correction of the data acquisition program
was essential because a negative baseline shift caused by
imbalance between the columns during the temperature
program would affect the recorded peak heights and could
not be detected on either the chart recorder or the computer.

Any deviations from normal peak retention times were investigated and corrected on a daily basis. Pyrolysis products were separated on a 1.5m by 4mm i.d. glass column packed with CAW (80-100 mesh) coated with 10% FFAP (Pye-Unicam). This was used in preference to the more usual Carbowax 20M because of its higher thermal stability. The packing extended only to the base of the injector oven, to prevent pyrolysis of the liquid phase and was held in place by a tight wad of silica thread. After each analysis, the column oven temperature was raised to 230°C for 10min to remove high boiling-point pyrolysis products before cooling to 80°C for the next analysis. The first six peaks were very high and were ignored. The chart recorder speed was 10mm/min with a sensitivity of 10mV. After 100 analyses, the column was removed, the inner wall in the injection area was cleaned and the top 5cm of packing replaced. The first three analyses after this procedure were not used and a test of pyrogram reproducibility was made.

Numerical analysis of data and identification program. A database comprising replicate pyrograms from each of 21 strains of Mobiluncus was collected and subjected to numerical analysis. Peak heights were normalised i.e. converted to percentages of the mean peak height of the 41 peaks for each pyrogram to correct for the amount of specimen pyrolysed (10). Total peak height over a selected set of peaks is commonly used as a correction factor (13). This approach is based on the assumption that all peaks are affected proportionally by variation in specimen weight although there appears to be no proof of this assumption in published work (14). Normalised peak heights (NPH's) were used in all subsequent calculations. Pyrograms were classified using CLUSTAN 1C (28) on an ICL

1906S mainframe computer. NPH's were scaled, dividing
each by the mean within replicate peak height variance, in
order to weight the peaks according to their replicate
reproducibility. Each pyrogram can be represented as a
point in multi-dimensional space (13), each of the 41 axes
corresponding to one of the observed peaks. Factor analysis
reduced this to an arbitrary 16 dimensions retaining the
distance structure. Euclidian distance in these 16 dimensions was used as a measure of dissimilarity between two
pyrograms and data was sorted into groups using heirarchical
unweighted pair group mean association (UPGMA). The multi-
variate statistical technique of discriminant analysis
using the S.P.S.S. subprogram "Discriminant" (17) run on a
Prime 750 minicomputer was used to produce a mathematical
identification system for pyrograms of unnamed isolates.
The NPH data for the selected peaks from the replicates of
the named isolates were the database. Using the discriminant
functions produced by this program, the computer printed
the likelihood of each isolate being a member of each of
the species.

RESULTS

Biochemistry and morphology. Using morphological and
biochemical parameters, the vaginosis associated anaerobic
curved rods could be divided into two main groups (Figure
1). Group I comprised short, comma-shaped, Gram-variable
organisms which had little saccharolytic activity. Group
II comprised long, Gram-negative curved rods which were
able to ferment a wide range of carbohydrates. Other
differential tests are shown in Table 1. In agreement
with other workers (22,24), each group could be subdivided.
Sub-group Ia (*M.curtisii* ss. *curtisii*) and Ib (*M.curtisii*
ss. *holmesii*) were morphologically indistinguishable as

Table 1. Differential Characters of *Mobiluncus* species.

Character	Group					Total nos. conforming
	Ia (8)	Ib (16)	IIa (20)	IIb (5)	III (1)	(50)
Length:width > 5	0	0	20	5	0	25
Yellow colonies	0	0	20	5	0	25
Retain Gram stain	8	16	0	0	1	25
Brown pigmentation (CBA)	0	0	13	2	0	15
haemolysis (CBA)	2	8	4	1	0	15
ONPG	8	16	0	0	1	25
Ammonia from arginine	8	15	0	0	1	24
Hippurate hydrolysis	8	16	0	0	1	25
Nitrate reduction	0	16	2	2	0	17
Metronidazole MIC > 8mg/l	8	16	12	4	1	41
Acid from:-						
D-Glucose	5	13	16	2	1	37
Sucrose	0	1	16	1	1	19
Raffinose	6	1	5	0	1	13
Lactose	0	0	5	0	0	5
meso-Inositol	0	0	15	0	0	15
D(+)Xylose	1	0	18	0	0	19
D(-)Ribose	0	1	18	0	1	20
D(+)Melezitose	0	0	8	0	1	9
D(+)Melibiose	8	1	4	0	1	14
D(+)Mannose	5	1	11	1	1	19
D(-)Fructose	3	5	17	1	1	27
Sorbitol	0	0	6	0	1	7
Maltose	7	6	19	0	1	33
D(+)Galactose	8	1	15	0	1	25
-methyl-D(+)-glucoside	2	2	16	0	1	21
N-acetyl-D(+)-glucosamine	0	0	11	0	1	12
Oyster glycogen	3	3	17	2	1	26
D(-)Arabinose	0	0	13	0	1	14

Strains AVA265 (Phillips);LCR (Sprott) and A99/83 (Skarin) clustered
in Group IIa. Strains AV50.7 (Phillips); SCR (Sprott) and A98/83
(Skarin) clustered in Group Ib.

were subgroups IIa and IIb (*M.mulieris*). Organisms in
sub-group Ia failed to reduce nitrate whereas those in
sub-group Ib produced nitrite from nitrate. Organisms in
sub-group IIa were able to ferment a wider range of carbohydrates than those in sub-group IIb. Further studies are
required to determine whether these constitute significant
differences. On further investigation, the organism in Group
III proved to be a mixed culture of *M. mulieris* and *M.curtisii*.

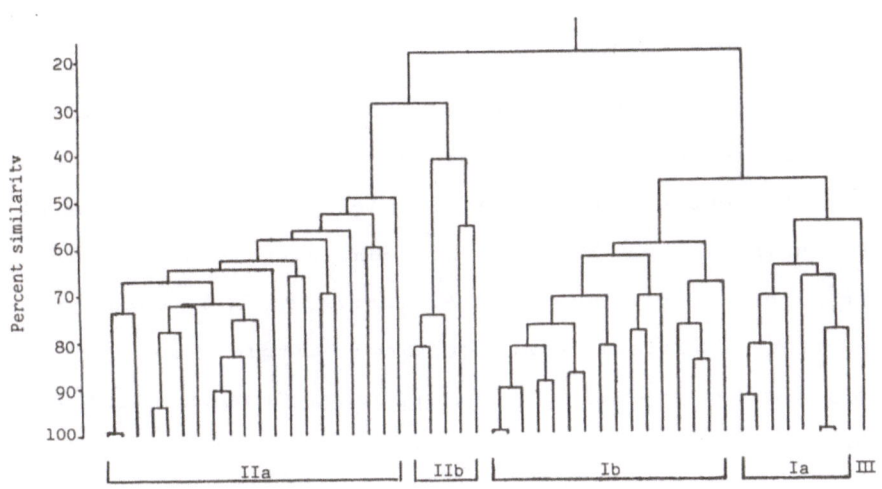

Figure 1. Dendrogram prepared by Jaccard Coefficient using 28 morphological and biochemical characters of 50 *Mobiluncus* strains. Ia, *M. curtisii* ss. *curtisii*; Ib, *M. curtisii* ss. *holmesii*; IIa and IIb, *M. mulieris*.

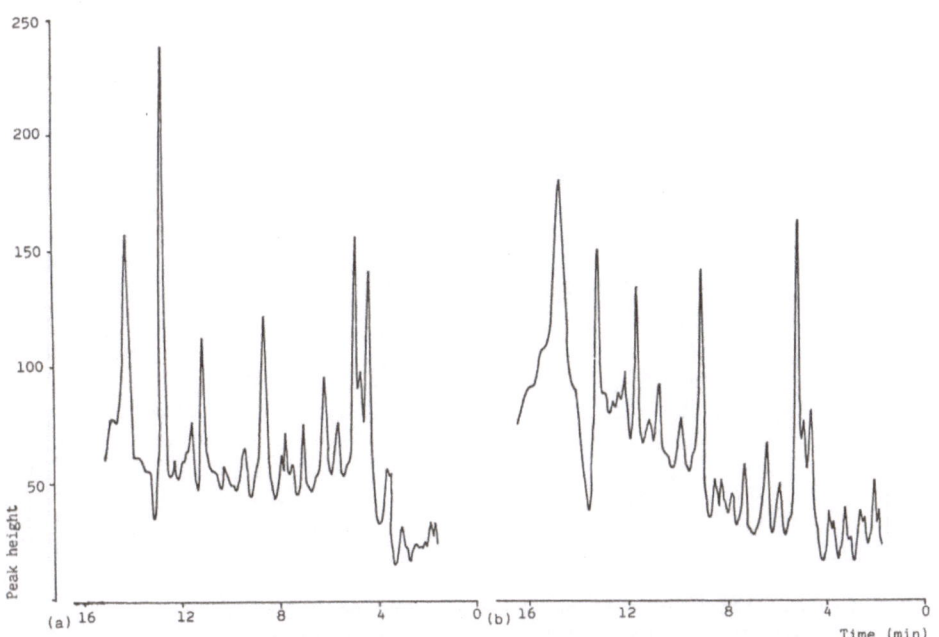

Figure 2. Typical pyrograms for (a) *Mobilincus curtisii* and (b) *M.mulieris*. Pyrolysis was started at time 0 min.

224

Pyrolysis. Typical pyrograms produced by *M. mulieris* and *M.curtisii* are shown in Figure 2. The two variants produce visually similar pyrograms, each with 41 peaks, illustrating the need for computer analysis of data. Principal components analysis obtains successive axes to illustrate maximal variation among the samples. The first and second principal components account for maximal variation and Figure 3 shows a two-dimensional plot of the clustering of like samples and distance between dissimilar samples. Strains of *M. mulieris* and *M. curtisii* fall into well separated clusters distinct from single isolates of *Campylobacter jejuni*, *C. fetus* ss. *fetus*, *Bacteroides ureolyticus*, *Vibrio cholerae*, *Gardnerella vaginalis* and *Haemophilus influenzae*. The classification of *Mobiluncus* spp. according to PGLC data is shown in Figure 4. The two species, although similar, are distinct from each other and from

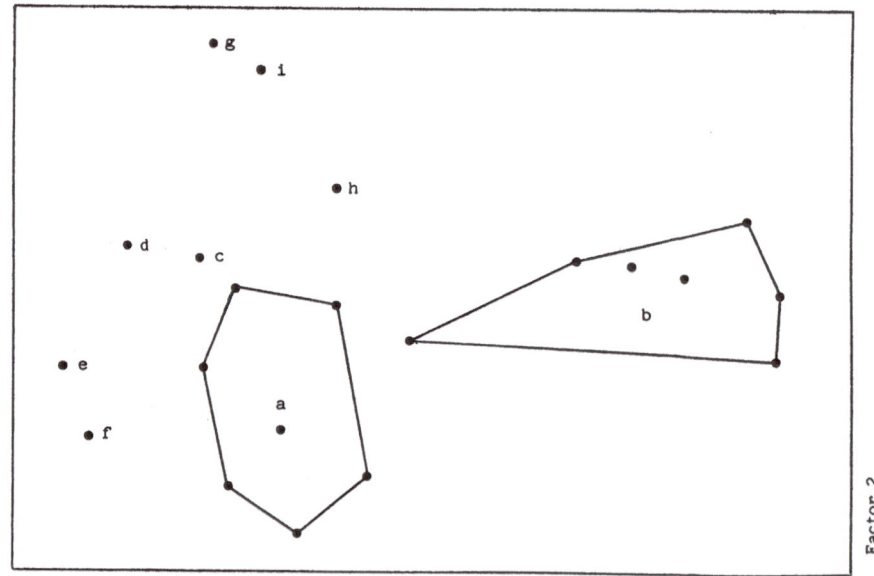

Figure 3. Plot representing the first and second principal components of PGLC data for: a, *Mobiluncus curtisii*; b, *M.mulieris*; c, *Campylobacter fetus* ss. *fetus*; d, *Bacteroides ureolyticus*; e and f, *C. jejuni*; g, *Vibrio cholerae*; h, *Gardnerella vaginalis* and i, *Haemophilus influenzae*. Column 2.

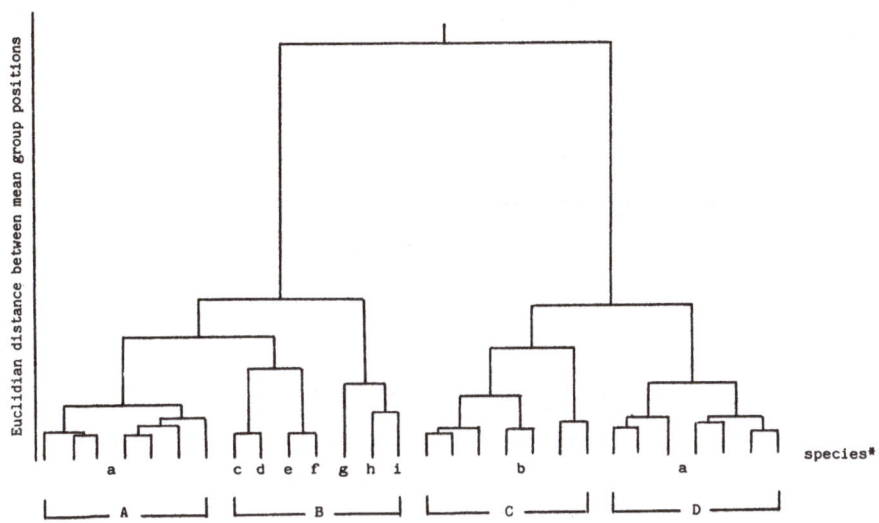

Figure 4. Dendrogram of 21 strains of *Mobiluncus* showing their relationship to each-other and to strains of other genera based upon PGLC data. a, *M. curtisii*; b, *M. mulieris*; c, *Campylobacter fetus* ss. *fetus*; d, *Bacteroides ureolyticus*; e and f, *C. jejuni*; g, *Vibrio cholerae*; h, *Gardnerella vaginalis* and i, *Haemophilus influenzae*. *Identification based upon biochemical tests. A, column 1; B,C, and D, column 2.

the reference strains. The organisms in Cluster A, although biochemically and morphologically similar to those in Cluster D, were pyrolysed on a different column using different methods to transfer colonies from plate to wire. A database of pyrograms of 30 strains of Mobiluncus with equal numbers from each species was subjected to discriminant analysis. This identified and printed appropriate weightings for each peak contributing significantly to discrimination between the species of *Mobiluncus*. Calculations using these factor weightings allowed subsequent assignment of an unknown pyrogram to species. The assignment of 30 strains of *Mobiluncus* to species on the basis of PGLC was in full agreement with identification by morphology and biochemistry.

DISCUSSION

Mobiluncus species are distinct from other known bacteria in morphology and biochemistry (19), in DNA base composition (27) and in SDS-PAGE peptide patterns (1). This distinctiveness is corroborated by the PGLC data reported here. PGLC of *Mobiluncus* spp. yielded two visually distinct but similar pyrogram patterns. Cluster analysis of the quantitative PGLC data revealed two distinct groups which corresponded to the two clusters of *M. mulieris* and *M. curtisii* obtained from numerical analysis of biochemical data. Strains characteristic of other genera did not enter either of these clusters. The use of discriminant analysis on a data-base comprising equal numbers of each species yielded correct identification of 30 strains of *Mobiluncus* species. Whole cell analysis of the genus *Mobiluncus* thus permitted rapid identification to species level. *M. curtisii* has been divided, tentatively, into two sub-species on the basis of nitrate reduction and migration through soft agar (24) although, on the basis of structural and biochemical data, other workers (5) did not subdivide this group. Sub-species of *M. curtisii* were not distinguished by double immunodiffusion and immunoblotting (21) or by SDS-PAGE (1). Although DNA hybridisation tests of *M. curtisii* indicated heterogeneity, sub-species could not be distinguished (5). The differentiation of sub-groups of *Mobiluncus* species by PGLC was beyond the ambit of this study and provides an area for further work. PGLC is technically difficult and has a low throughput because of serial processing. Although inter-column reproducibility is low, column degradation may be delayed by the use of a liquid phase with a high thermal stability (14). The technique is rapid (analysis times of 30 minutes); objective; allows complete automation (15); produces a novel type of data for taxonomic studies and reflects the overall composition of the organism. We found that complex preparation of bacterial cultures prior to identification by PGLC was unnecessary. Despite the difficulty of the technique, PGLC can be used successfully in the identification of strains of a group of related species. The introduction of PGLC as a routine identification technique is hindered by problems in inter-column and inter-apparatus reproducibility but these may be overcome by the use of pyrolysis-mass-spectrometry.

ACKNOWLEDGEMENTS

The authors wish to acknowledge Professor I. Phillips (Dept. of Microbiology, St.Thomas Hospital, London, SE1 7EH), Dr M.S. Sprott (Regional Public Health Laboratory, Newcastle upon Tyne, NE4 6BE) and Dr A. Skarin (Dept. of Medical Microbiology, University of Lund, Solvegatand 23, 223 62 Lund, Sweden) for kindly providing strains. We would also like to thank Dr R.C. Spencer for assisting with the preparation of this manuscript.

References

1   Baron, E.J., Wexler. H.M. and Finegold. S.M.   1984.
     Biochemical and polyacrylamide gel electrophoretic
     analyses of vaginosis associated anaerobic curved
     rods.   In: P-A.Mardh and D.Taylor-Robinson (eds.).
     Bacterial Vaginosis.   Almqvist & Wiksell International
     Stockholm, Sweden, pp.65-69.

2   Blackwell, A.L. and Barlow, D.   1982.   Clinical
     diagnosis of anaerobic vaginosis.
     Br. J. Venereal Dis. 58: 387-393.

3   Blackwell, A.L., Fox, A.R., Phillips, I. and Barlow,D.
     1983.   Anaerobic vaginosis: clinical, microbiological
     and therapeutic findings.   Lancet. 2: 1379-82.

4   Buhler, C. and Simon, W. 1970.   Curie-point pyrolysis
     gas chromatography.
     J. Chromatographic Sci.   8: 323-329.

5   Christiansen, G., Hansen, E., Holst, E., Christiansen,
     C. and Mardh, P-A.   1984.   Genetic relationships of
     short and long anaerobic curved rods isolated from the
     vagina.   In: P-A. Mårdh and D. Taylor-Robinson (eds.).
     Bacterial Vaginosis.   Almqvist & Wiksell International
     Stockholm, Sweden, pp.75-78.

6   Curtis, A.H. 1913.   A motile curved anaerobic bacillus
     in uterine discharges.   J. Infectious Dis. 12: 165-169.

7   Drucker, D.B.   1976.   Gas-liquid chromatographic
     chemotaxonomy.   In: J.R. Norris (ed.).   Methods in
     microbiology, vol 9.   Academic Press, London, pp.51-
     125.

8   Durieux, R. and Dublanchet, A.   1980.   Les "vibrions"
     anaerobies des leucorrhees.   Technique d'isolement et
     sensibilite aux antibiotiques.
     Medicine et Maladies Infectieuses, 10: 109-115.

9   Glupczynski, Y., Labbe, M., Crokaert, F., Pepersack,
     F., van der Auwera, P. and Yourassowsky, E.   1984.
     Isolation of *Mobiluncus* in four cases of extragenital
     infections in adult women.
     Eur. J. Clin. Microbiol. 3: 433-435.

10   Gutteridge, C.S. and Norris, J.R.   1979.   The
     application of pyrolysis techniques to the
     identification of micro-organisms.
     J. Appl. Bacteriol. 47: 5-43.

11   Kronig, I. 1895.   Uber die Natur der Scheidenkeime,
     speciell uber das Vorkommen anaerober Streptokokken im
     Scheidensekret Schwangerer.
     Zentralbl Gynakol, 19: 409-412.

12   Levett, P.N.   1984.   Development and evaluation of a
     miniaturised method as an aid to the identification of
     clinically important anaerobic bacteria.
     J. Clin. Path. 37: 70-73.

13 MacFie, J.H., Gutteridge, C.S. and Norris, J.R. 1978.
    Use of canonical variates analysis in differentiation
    of bacteria by pyrolysis gas-liquid chromatography.
    J. Gen. Microbiol. 104: 67-74.

14 Magee, J.T., Hindmarch, J.M. and Meechan, D.F. 1983.
    Identification of *staphylococci* by pyrolysis gas-
    liquid chromatography.
    J. Med. Microbiol. 16: 483-495.

15 Meuzelaar, H.L., Kistemaker, P.G. and Tom, A. 1975.
    Rapid and automated identification of micro-organisms
    by Curie-point pyrolysis techniques, I.
    Differentiation of bacterial strains by fully
    automated Curie-point pyrolysis gas-liquid
    chromatography. In: C.G. Heden and T. Illeni (eds.).
    New approaches to the identification of micro-
    organisms. John Wiley and Sons, New York, pp.165-178.

16 Moi, H., Schoenknecht, F., Tornqvist, E. and
    Danielsson, D. 1984. A serological study of
    anaerobic curved rods with rabbit hyperimmune
    antisera. In: P-A.Mårdh and D.Taylor-Robinson (eds.).
    Bacterial Vaginosis. Almqvist & Wiksell International
    Stockholm, Sweden, pp.79-85.

17 Nie, N.H., Hull, C.H., Jenkin, J.G., Steinbrenner, K.
    and Bent, D.H. 1975. Statistical Package for the
    Social Sciences, McGraw-Hill, New York.

18 Pahlson, C., Forsum, U., Hallen, A., Hjelm, E. and
    Wallin, J. 1983. Characterisation of motile
    anaerobic curved rods isolated from women with lower
    genital tract infection in three different countries.
    Eur. J. Sex. Trans. Dis. 1: 73-75.

19 Pahlson, C., Bergqvist, F. and Forsum, U. 1984.
    Numerical taxonomy of motile anaerobic curved rods
    isolated from vaginal discharge. In: P-A. Mårdh and
    D. Taylor-Robinson (eds.). Bacterial Vaginosis.
    Almqvist & Wiksell International Stockholm, Sweden,
    pp.251-256.

20 Phillips, I. and Taylor, E. 1982. Anaerobic curved
    rods in vaginitis. Lancet, 1: 221.

21 Roberts, M.C., Baron, E.J., Finegold, S.M. and Kenny,
    G.E. 1985. Antigenic distinctiveness of *Mobiluncus
    curtisii* and *Mobiluncus mulieris*.
    J. Clin. Microbiol. 21: 891-893.

22 Spiegel, C.A. 1983. Further characterisation of
    curved motile anaerobic bacteria associated with
    bacterial vaginosis. In: Abstracts, 83rd Annual
    Meeting, American Society for Microbiology, C289.

23 Spiegel,C.A., Eschenbach,D.A., Amsel,R. and
    Holmes,K.K. 1983. Curved anaerobic bacteria in
    bacterial vaginosis and their response to
    antimicrobial therapy.
    J. Infect. Dis. 148: 817-822.

24 Spiegel, C.A. and Roberts, M. 1984. *Mobiluncus*
    gen.nov., *Mobiluncus curtisii* subsp. *curtisii* sp.nov.,
    Mobiluncus curtisii subsp. *holmesii* subsp.nov. and
    Mobiluncus mulieris sp.nov., curved rods from the
    human vagina. Int. J. Syst. Bacteriol. 34: 177-184.

25 Sprott,M.S., Ingham, H.R., Pattman, R.S., Eisenstadt,
    R.L., Short, G.R., Narang, H.K., Sisson, P.R. and
    Selkon, J.B. 1983. Characteristics of motile curved
    rods in vaginal secretions.
    J. Med. Microbiol. 16: 175-182.

26 Sturm, A.W. and Sikkenk, P.J. 1984. Anaerobic curved
    rods in breast abscess. Lancet, 2: 1216.

27 Taylor, A.J. and Owen, R.J. 1984. Morphological and
    chemical characteristics of anaerobic curved rod-
    shaped bacteria from the female genital tract. In: P-
    A. Mårdh and D. Taylor-Robinson (eds.). Bacterial
    Vaginosis. Almqvist & Wiksell International
    Stockholm, Sweden, pp.97-106.

28 Wishart, D. 1978. The CLUSTAN user manual. 3rd
    edition. Inter-university/research council series.
    Report No47 (Jan).

CHAPTER 20

ANAEROBES IN NON-GONOCOCCAL URETHRITIS, BALANOPOSIHITIS AND GENITAL ULCERS

B. I. Duerden

Medical Microbiology Department, University of Sheffield
Medical School, Beech Hill Road, Sheffield, S10 2RX, U.K.

Contents

Introduction

Anaerobic Genito-Urinary infections in men

      Balanoposthitis and NGU

      Genital Ulcers

      Urethritis

Conclusion

References

INTRODUCTION

The genitalia are no exception to the general anaerobic colonisation of the human body. They are in fact a very fruitful area of study for the anaerobic bacteriologist. As is shown in the preceding papers, a great deal of time and effort has been devoted to the study of the female genital flora (2,12), but less attention has been paid to the male.

There is still some debate about the place of *Bacteroides* and other anaerobes in the normal flora of men; there is only a little hard evidence yet but it seems likely that anaerobes other than the skin propionibacteria or coryneforms contribute only a relatively small part of the normal flora. This seems fairly certain for *Bacteroides* – a little less sure for anaerobic cocci. In one of our recent studies (7) we collected urethral swabs from men with balanoposthitis or urethritis and from healthy controls. In the 28 controls, the flora was predominantly aerobic. Anaerobes were found in only six (21%) and only four had *Bacteroides* spp. – a very different picture from the patient groups that are described below. Fontaine and his colleagues at the Clinical Research Centre had slightly different findings (5); they found anaerobes in 80% of controls. This high rate was due almost entirely to anaerobic Gram-positive cocci in the anterior urethra of 67% of normal males; Gram-negative anaerobic bacilli were uncommon (in 27% of subjects) and in small numbers, as in our study. Therefore, bacteroides do not seem to be a normal, major feature in man.

Although data on the normal flora are scanty, there is plenty of evidence that anaerobes are involved in infections in men, particularly superficial infections of the genitalia that can be very severe and destructive. Such conditions as balanoposthitis, superficial abscesses, and scrotal or inguinal gangrene are, in general, anaerobic infections. They are not necessarily caused by one pathogen, but more probably by a mixture of anaerobes and, possibly, facultative species (1, 3, 7, 8). The severity of some of these synergistic bacterial gangrenes has been recognised since the earliest descriptions by Meleney (9) and Fournier (10), but less florid forms of these conditions are common. There is also the question of non-gonococcal (non-specific) urethritis (NGU). Chlamydia are important but are by no means the whole answer. Are anaerobes involved here?

ANAEROBIC GENITO-URINARY INFECTIONS IN MEN

The basic questions we need to ask in relation to any of these conditions are:

- are anaerobes primary pathogens?

- do they contribute to synergistic infections?

- if so, which species have a pathogenic role?

In this paper I will consider these questions by drawing on our experience in Sheffield during the last few years and coupling that with the work of the team at the Clinical Research Centre. We had been working initially on bacterial vaginosis and because of the problems of relapse or reinfection in women, we looked at a group of men to see whether their NGU or balanitis might be related to vaginosis. That is still not entirely clear but the results were interesting and took us in other directions. Balanoposthitis and NGU. In the earliest study we examined a group of men with balanoposthitis; in 68 men, *Gardnerella vaginalis* was found in only 23 but *Bacteroides* spp. in 60. There were 15 with a mixture of the two, eight with *G. vaginalis* only, but 45 yielded bacteroides without *G. vaginalis*. The *Bacteroides* spp. included asaccharolytic species, known to be involved in necrotising infections (3) and members of the melaninogenicus-oralis groups generally recognised to be vaginal organisms (2). The findings suggested that bacteroides may play a prominent role in this condition. We then looked at the

Table 1. Anaerobes from men with balanoposthitis and/or NGU.

Species		Number of isolates
Bacteroides		115
Asaccharolytic group	58	
B. asaccharolyticus		42
B. ureolyticus		16
Melaninogenicus–oralis group	57	
B. melaninogenicus		8
B. intermedius		17
B. levi		2
B. bivius		16
B. disiens		7
B. oralis		7
Anaerobic cocci		33
Clostridia		3
Bifidobacteria		1
TOTAL		152

question of *Bacteroides* spp. in normal controls and two groups of patients, one with urethritis and the other with balanitis or balanoposthitis (7). We examined urethral and sub-preputial swabs from 150 men. The findings with the two swabs were similar and the results have been combined. The series included 28 asymptomatic controls with no signs of genital disease, 24 with NGU alone, 79 with balanitis or balanoposthitis and 19 with balanoposthitis and NGU.

In the 28 controls, as described above, the flora was predominantly aerobic; anaerobes were found in only six (21%) and only four had *Bacteroides*. They were found, however, in most of the patients in all three disease groups – 60 (76%) with balanoposthitis alone, 16 (67%) with NGU alone and 18 (75%) with both conditions. Each of these figures is highly significant when compared with the controls. Not only were anaerobes present in many cases but when they were present they were the predominant microbial flora – and bacteroides were the commonest species. *Bacteroides* were found in 84 (89%) of the 94 patients with anaerobes. Of 152 strains of anaerobic bacteria isolated, there were 115 *Bacteroides* strains (Table 1). The melaninogenicus-oralis and asaccharolytic groups were both represented; *B. asaccharolyticus* was the commonest single species followed by *B. intermedius, B. ureolyticus* and *B. bivius*. Most of the others were Gram-positive non-sporing anaerobes, mostly anaerobic cocci. Clostridia had no significant role.

B. ureolyticus is interesting. It was isolated from five of 14 men with erosive balanoposthitis (36%) but only eight (10%) of 82 men with non-erosive disease. The combination of *B. asaccharolyticus* and *B. ureolyticus* was also highest in erosive balanoposthitis – although numbers were very small. This all suggested that anaerobes

especially *Bacteroides*, might be important - as in other
necrotising and putrid lesions. We then pursued the two
conditions, urethritis and ulceration, in separate studies.
<u>Genital Ulcers</u>. We studied the bacteriology of genital
ulcers by examining swabs from 91 patients (46 male and 45
female). We concentrated particularly upon the role of
herpes simplex virus, *Haemophilus ducreyi* and anaerobes,
although we did general bacteriological cultures as well
(8).

There were no cases of syphilis, but herpes simplex
virus was isolated from 52 (57%) patients, and *H. ducreyi*
from 12 (13%). In 27 (30%) none of these established
pathogens was isolated.

In the control males studied previously, the predominant flora had been aerobic; now the predominance of
anaerobes in ulcers in men was highly significant. The
results obtained with women with ulcers were the same -
again, anaerobes predominated in ulcer patients. Not only
were anaerobes present, they formed the major part of the
cultivable flora and it was the *Bacteroides* spp. that were

Table 2. Anaerobes from genital ulcers.

| Species | Number of subjects with the given species | | |
	Controls (male) (n = 24)	Ulcer patients male (n = 46)	female (n = 45)
Bacteroides	3	30	35
Asaccharolytic group	2	26	21
B. asaccharolyticus	2	23	15
B. ureolyticus	0	26	15
Melaninogenicus-oralis group	1	10	23
Anaerobic cocci	2	10	15

isolated significantly more frequently in ulcer patients (Table 2). In men this difference was accounted for entirely by the isolation rates of the asaccharolytic bacteroides – *B.asaccharolyticus* and *B.ureolyticus* (there were no significant differences between controls and patients for other anaerobes). In women, the asaccharolytic species were again common, but there were also high isolation rates of the oralis – melaninogenicus group.

When we examined the relationship between herpes simplex virus and bacteria, the isolation rates (percentages) of anaerobes (and aerobes for that matter) were the same from herpetic and non-herpetic ulcers (Table 3). The only difference was with *Candida albicans*, which was isolated only from non-herpetic ulcers. The interaction

Table 3. Bacterial flora of herpetic and non-herpetic ulcers

Species	Percentage of ulcers colonised	
	HSV +ve (n = 52)	HSV –ve (n = 39)
H. ducreyi	18	10
Other aerobes	67	65
C. albicans	6	31
Bacteroides spp.	64	77
Asaccharolytic group	46	56
Melaninogenicus–oralis group	28	42
Other anaerobes	26	35

HSV = herpes simplex virus

between virus and bacteria is not clear. I do not doubt the significance of herpes simplex virus, at least as an initiator of acute superficial, tender ulcers. However, anaerobic superinfection of the damaged epithelium causing more extensive damage could be responsible for the deeper, phagedenic ulcers with necrotic bases that are typical of more long-standing lesions.

The large proportion of patients in the erosive balanoposthitis and genital ulcer groups with anaerobes and the contribution of *B.asaccharolyticus* and *B.ureolyticus* relates very closely to our other work with these species in which both appeared to be significant pathogens in superficial, necrotising lesions - decubitis and varicose ulcers, diabetic gangrene and perineal lesions, including those that would be well described as synergistic gangrene (3,4).

I think that there can be little doubt that these anaerobes are significant pathogens in ulcerative genital lesions, although not necessarily as primary or sole pathogens. The relationship with herpes simplex virus infection needs further study.

Urethritis. Our initial findings in patients with NGU (see above) stimulated further extensive studies of the microbial flora in urethritis. This had also been pursued by Fontaine and his colleagues at the Clinical Research Centre. Our results are not yet available, because the specimen code has not yet been broken to separate controls from patients. However, even at this stage it is clear that there are two patterns of results: one set of speci-mens with little variation - coagulase negative staphylococci and diphtheroids (aerobic and anaerobic) and little else; and a second set with much greater variety and with large numbers of anaerobes, particularly *Bacteroides*. This could well fit the pattern of our previous study (7) in which patients with urethritis had a gross excess of anaerobes, mostly *Bacteroides*, in urethral cultures. This does not necessarily mean that they are a primary cause of urethritis, but they may be and Fontaine

Table 4. Isolation of *B. ureolyticus* from men with NGU

Patient group			Number examined	*B. ureolyticus* isolated (%)
NGU	–	all	64	32 (50)
	–	Chlamydia negative	50	28 (56)
	–	Chlamydia and Ureoplasma negative	31	19 (61)
Gonorrhoea			7	1 (14)
Controls			30	4 (13)

Fontaine et al., 1983 (5,6)

et al. (5,6) have found a Gram-negative anaerobic bacillus with a clear association with urethritis and have suggested that it may be a specific cause. In their study it was present as the predominant organism in urethral specimens from 50% of 64 men with NGU (Table 4). The figures were 56% for chlamydia-negative and 61% for chlamydia – and ureoplasma-negative patients. It was rarely found in 30 controls without NGU. The identity of this organism has now been confirmed as *B. ureolyticus* by Taylor and his colleagues at the National Collection of Type Cultures, Colindale, London (11).

We have not been able to confirm this in our patients – we have only a few *B. ureolyticus* isolates and most of our *Bacteroides* are *bivius*, *disiens*, *melaninogenicus* and *asaccharolyticus*. I am not sure of the explanation of all this.   The only conclusion I can draw is that *Bacteroides* are   there   - their presence indicates that   something   is wrong.   They may be the cause of the disease, or they may be secondary pathogens,   or they may just be indicators of abnormality,   colonising   a damaged mucosa,   although   the idea   of   a harmless bacteroides   under   these   conditions seems a little unlikely.

CONCLUSION

Is there a pattern emerging? Possibly.   In the normal man   anaerobes may be a relatively minor component of   the urethral and genital flora; anaerobic cocci may be present but bacteroides do not make a major contribution. However, in   ulcerative and erosive lesions the   evidence   supports the   hypothesis   of   anaerobic   pathogenicity   and   in urethritis   there   may   be some role   for   the   anaerobes. There   is   enough   evidence   for   microbiologists   to   be interested in this area but there is still a great deal to be discovered.

References

1   Chapel, T., Brown, W.J., Jeffries, C. and Stewart, J.A. 1978. The microbiological flora of penile ulcerations. J. Infect. Dis. 137: 50-6.

2   Duerden, B.I. 1980. The isolation and identification of *Bacteroides* spp. from the normal human vaginal flora. J. Med. Microbiol. 13: 79-87.

3   Duerden, B.I. 1980. The identification of Gram-negative anaerobic bacilli isolated from clinical infections. J. Hyg. (Camb.) 84: 301-13.

4   Duerden, B.I., Bennett, K.W. and Faulkner, J. 1982. Isolation of *Bacteroides ureolyticus* (*B. corrodens*) from clinical infections. J. Clin. Pathol. 35: 309-12.

5   Fontaine, E.A.R., Taylor-Robinson, D., Hanna, N.F., and Coufalik, E.D. 1982. Anaerobes in men with urethritis. Br. J. Vener. Dis. 58: 321-6.

6   Fontaine, E.A.R., Borriello, S.P., Taylor-Robinson, D. and Davies, H.A. 1984. Characteristics of a Gram-negative anaerobe isolated from men with non-gonococcal urethritis. J. Med. Microbiol. 17: 129-40.

7   Masfari, A.N., Kinghorn, G.R. and Duerden, B.I. 1983. Anaerobes in genito-urinary infections in men. Br. J. Vener. Dis. 59: 255-9.

8   Masfari, A.N., Kinghorn, G.R., Hafiz, S., Barton, I.G. and Duerden, B.I. 1985. Anaerobic bacteria and herpes simplex virus in genital ulceration. Genitourin. Med. 61: 109-13.

9   Meleney, F.L. 1933. A differential diagnosis between certain types of infectious gangrene of the skin: with particular reference to haemolytic streptococcus gangrene and bacterial synergistic gangrene. Surg. Gynecol. Obstet. 56: 847-67.

10   Randall A. 1920. Idiopathic gangrene of the scrotum. J. Ureol. 4 : 219-35.

11   Taylor, A.J., Dawson, C.A. and Owen, R.J. The identification of *Bacteroides ureolyticus* from patients with non-gonococcal urethritis by conventional biochemical tests and by DNA and protein analysis. J. Med. Microbiol. (in press).

12   Wilks, M.N., Thin, R.N. and Tabaqchali, S. 1982. Quantitative methods for studies on vaginal flora. J. Med. Microbiol. 15: 141-7.

Chairman of session : Dr. J.M. Hardie

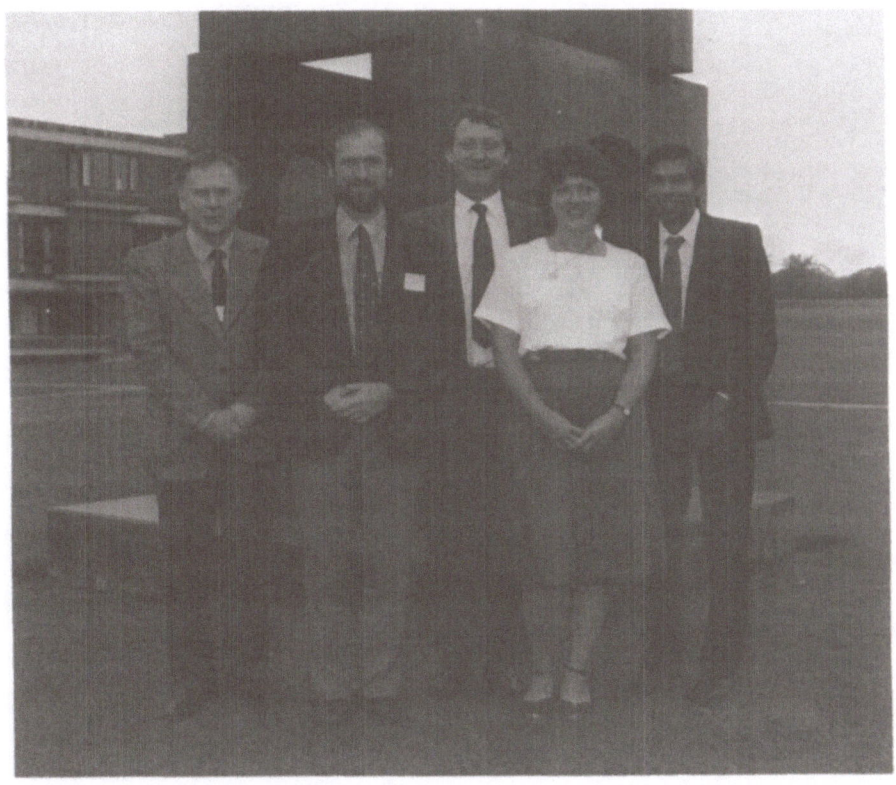

From left to right :

W.D. Grant, J.M.Hardie, R.J. Carman, Elizabeth A. Taylor and H.N.Shah

CHAPTER 21

ANAEROBIC ARCHAEBACTERIA

W.D. Grant

Department of Microbiology, University of Leicester, Leicester, LE1 7RH, UK.

Contents

An introduction to Archaebacteria

References

AN INTRODUCTION TO ARCHAEBACTERIA

The archaebacteria comprise several distinct phenotypes including extreme halophiles, certain thermophiles
and the methanogens. Despite the phenotypic diversity of
the group as a whole, partial sequence analyses of 16S
rRNA by Woese and colleagues (1,2) have indicated that
these prokaryotes represent a well-defined third line of
evolutionary descent different from all other prokaryotes
(the eubacteria) and the eukaryotic line. There is now a
wealth of additional biochemical detail supporting the
separate evolutionary lineage of the group including the
nature of archaebacterial cell walls (which lack peptidoglycan) and major differences in transcriptional and
translation equipment (3,4). In particular, unlike
eubacteria and eukaryotes, archaebacteria have membranes
based on ether-linked isopranyl core lipids (5). In the
majority of cases these lipids are $C_{20}C_{20}$ glycerol
biphytanyl diethers or $C_{40}C_{40}$ dibiphytanyl diglycerol
tetraethers, although certain halophiles are unusual in
possessing sesterterpanyl (C_{25}) chains as well as C_{20}
chains in ether linkage to glycerol (6).

Detailed nucleic acid analyses indicate that
archaebacteria have two main branches, the methanogens and
halophiles comprising one major group, and sulphur-
dependent thermophiles comprising the second main branch
(7). One particular thermophilic archaebacterium
Thermoplasma acidophilum does not appear to be closely
related to either branch. The methanogenic archaebacteria
and the sulphur-dependent arachaebacteria with the

exception of *Sulfolobus* spp. are all strict anaerobes. In recent times it has become clear that even *Sulfolobus* spp. are capable of anaerobic sulphur-dependent growth (8,9) as well as aerobic sulphur-dependent growth, and we have shown that those halophiles we have tested are also capable of anaerobic sulphur-dependent growth. It is of note that methanogens are also capable of sulphur reduction (10). *Thermoplasma acidophilum* has not been tested in this respect, but it is likely then that anaerobic growth in the presence of sulphur is a general archaebacterial trait. Thus those archaebacteria that can also grow aerobically need not necessarily have evolved more recently (after the appearance of an aerobic atmosphere).

Sulphur-dependent archaebacteria are in the main morphologically characteristic, making identification relatively straightforward. Temperature range and substrate utilization is also useful in this respect (II). The methanogens and halophiles on the other hand are rather uniform in morphology (with a few exceptions) and in substrate utilization (12) making these subgroups difficult to classify in detail except by applying sophisticated nucleic acid analyses. However, polar lipid analyses and core ether lipid analyses have proved valuable as more rapid indications of taxonomic status, and the groups so derived are consistent with groups derived from nucleic acid hybridization and sequencing studies (13,14).

References

1   Woese, C.R., Magrum, L.J. and Fox, G.E.   1978.
    Archaebacteria. J. Molec. Evol. 13:   73-83.

2   Woese, C.R. and Fox, G.E.   1977.   Phylogenetic
    structure of the   prokaryotic domain: The primary
    kingdoms.   Proc. Nat. Acad. Sci. (Wash.)   74: 5088-5090.

3   Woese, C.R.   1982.   Archaebacteria and cellular
    origins: An overview.
    Zbl. Bakt. Hyg. I. Abt. Orig.   C3:   1-17.

4   Woese, C.R.   1981.   Archaebacteria.
    Sci. Amer. 244: 89-122.

5   Langworthy, T.A. Tornabene, T.G. and Holzer, G.   1982.
    Lipids of archaebacteria.
    Zbl. Bakt. Hyg. I. Abt. Orig. C3: 228-244.

6   De Rosa, M., Gambacorta, A., Nicolaus, B. and Grant,
    W.D.   1982.   An assymetric archaebacterial diether
    lipid from alkaliphilic halophiles.
    J. Gen. Microbiol.   128:   343-348.

7   Woese, C.R., Gupta, R., Hahn, C.M., Zillig, W. and Tu,
    J.   1984.   The phylogenetic relationship of three
    sulphur dependent archaebacteria.   Nature   313: 787-789.

8   Segerer, A., Stetter, O. and Klink, F.   1985.   Two
    contrary modes of chemolithotrophy in the same
    archaebacteria.   Nature   313:   787-789.

9   Zillig, W., Yeats, S., Holz, I., Bock, A., Grapp, F.,
    Rettenberger, M. and Lutz, S.   1985.   Plasmid-related
    anaerobic autotrophy of the novel archaebacterium
    Sulfolobus ambivilans. Nature   313:   789-791.

10 Stetter, O. and Gaag, G.   1983.   Reduction of
    molecular sulphur by   methogenic bacteria.
    Nature   305:   309-311.

11 Zillig, W., Holz, I., Janekovic, D., Schafer, W. and
    Reiter, W.D.   1983.   The archaebacterium
    Thermococcus celer represents a novel genus within the
    thermophilic bracnh of the archaebacteria.
    Syst. Appl. Microbiol.   4:   88-94.

12 Balch, W.E., Fox, G.E., Magrum, L.J., Woese, C.R. and
    Wolfe, R.S. 1979.   Methanogens: re-evaluation of a
    unique biological group. Microbiol. Rev.   43:   260-296.

13 Ross, H.N.M. and Grant W.D.   1985.   Nucleic acid
    studies on halophilic archaebacteria.
    J. Gen. Microbiol.   131: 165-173.

14 Ross, H.N.M., Grant, W.D. and Harris, J.E. 1985.
    Lipids in archaebacterial taxonomy.   In: Chemical
    Methods in Bacterial Systematics. (eds.) M. Goodfellow
    & D. Minnikin.   pp.289-300.   Academic Press.

CHAPTER 22

RECENT ADVANCES IN THE TAXONOMY OF THE GENUS *BACTEROIDES*

M.D. Collins and H.N. Shah[1]

Department of Food Microbiology, Food Research Institute, Shinfield, Reading, RG2 9AT, UK.

[1]Department of Oral Microbiology, London Hospital Medical College, Turner Street, London E1 2AD, UK.

Contents

Review

References

REVIEW

The genus *Bacteroides* as described in Bergey's Manual of Systematic Bacteriology (4) comprises a heterogeneous collection of obligately anaerobic Gram-negative non-sporeforming rod-shaped bacteria. Over forty species are currently recognised. These species are phenotypically very diverse and possess a DNA base composition range of 28-61 mol% G + C although it is now generally acepted that a difference of >10% indicates species are unrelated at the generic level (8). In addition to this wide range in DNA base composition, members of the genus exhibit a variety of cellular morphologies and are biochemically and physio-logically extremely heterogenous (8).

Over recent years the application of biochemical and chemical methods has done much to clarify the taxonomic interrelationships of members of the genus *Bacteroides*. On the basis of biochemical, chemical and genetic criteria it is now clear that the genus *Bacteroides* should be restricted to the "*Bacteroides fragilis* group" of org-anisms (viz. *B.fragilis*, *B.distasonis*, *B.thetaiotaomicron*, *B.eggerthii*, *B.ovatus*, *B.uniformis* and *B.vulgatus*). Members of the "*B.fragilis* group" are biochemically and chemically relatively homogeneous and facilitate a tighter definition of the genus. The genus *Bacteroides* sould be restricted to those species which:

a) are obligately anaerobic, Gram-negative non-sporeforming rods

b) produce major amounts of acetic and succinic acids (and lower levels of other acids)

c) contain malate dehydrogenase, glutamate dehydrogenase, glucose-6-phosphate dehydrogenase and 6-phosphogluconate dehydrogenase

d) possess a DNA base composition within the approximate
    limiting range of 40-48 mol% G + C

e) possess sphingolipids

f) possess predominantly straight-chain saturated,
    anteiso-methyl branched and *iso*-methyl branched
    long-chain fatty acids

g) contain menaquinones (major components MK-10, M-11).

Species conforming to this definition are given in
Table 1.

Using the above criteria species which possess relatively high mol% G + C values (e.g. *B.multiacidus* 56-58
mol%, *B.microfuses* 60-61%, *B.capillosus* 60%) can be
readily excluded from the genus. *Bacteroides multiacidus*
and *B.microfusus* have recently been classified in two new
genera as *Mitsuokella multiacidus* (7) and *Rikenella
microfusus* (3) respectively. *Bacteroides* capillosus
shares little interspecies DNA homology with *M.multiacidus*
and *R. microfusus* and also warrants a new genus (Tables 1
& 2).

Species with DNA base compositions in the range 28 to
37 mol% should also be excluded from the genus *Bacteroides*.
B. hypermegas and *B. termitidis* are phenotypically quite
different from each other and all the other *Bacteroides*
(7, Shah & Collins 1983, 9, 2). On the basis of 16s-
ribosomal RNA cataloguing the latter species has also been
shown to be phylogenetically distinct from all defined
eubacterial 'phyla' (5). *Bacteroides hypermegas* and
B.termiditis have now been reclassified in two new genera,
as *Megamonas hypermegas* (6) and *Sebaldella termitidis* (8)
respectively. The biochemical and chemical characteristics
of the non- or very weakly fermentative species (viz:
B.coagulans, *B.furcosus*, *B.praeacutus*, *B.ureolyticus*)
whose DNA base compositions range between 28-37 mol% G+C

Table 1. Proposed taxonomic revision of the genus *Bacteroides*.

Species	Taxonomic status / Comments
"*B. fragilis* group" *B. fragilis, B. distasonis, B. eggerthii,* *B. ovatus, B. uniformis, B. vulgatus* *B. thetaiotaomicron*	Genus *Bacteroides*
"*B. oralis/melaninogenicus*" group *B. bivius, B. buccae, B. buccalis,* *B. denticola, B. intermedius, B. disiens* *B. loeschii, B. oralis, B. oulorum,* *B. oris, B. ruminicola, B. veroralis* *B. melaninogenicus, B. corporis,*	New genus
"Pigmented asaccharolytic group" *B. asaccharolyticus, B. endodontalis,* *B. gingivalis*	New genus
B. amylophilus	New genus
B. capillosus	New genus
B. coagulans	New genus
B. furcosus	*Anaerorhabdus*
B. gracilis	*Wolinella*
B. hypermegas	*Megamonas*
B. levii	Uncertain (possibly related to pigmented asaccharolytic group)
B. macacae	Uncertain (possibly related to pigmented asaccharolytic group)
B. microfusus	*Rikenella*
B. multiacidus	*Mitsuokella*
B. nodosus	Uncertain (not *Bacteroides*)
B. praecutus	New genus
B. putredinis	Uncertain (possibly related to *B. macacae* and pigmented asaccharolytic group).
B. polypragmatus	Uncertain (not *Bacteroides*)
B. pneumosintes	Uncertain (not *Bacteroides*)
B. splanchnicus	Uncertain (not *Bacteroides*)
B. succinogenes	New genus
B. termiditis	*Sebaldella*
B. ureolyticus	New genus
B. zoogleoformans	Uncertain

are also incompatible with their inclusion in the genus.
Although these non-fermentative organisms superficially
appear to form a homogeneous group of 'atypical bacteroides',
biochemical, chemical and genetic data indicate they are
taxonomically very diverse. Metabolic end products
(presumably in some cases derived from nitrogen metabolism)
vary widely amongst these species as do their dehydrogenase patterns and lipid composition (see table 3).
Bacteroides furcosus has recently been reclassified as
Anaerorhabdus furcosus (8). Although the remaining non-
fermentative species have not as yet been reclassified,
biochemical and chemical criteria indicate they probably

Table 2. Biochemical and Chemical characerics useful in the
differentiation of *Bacteroides capillosus*, *Mitsuokella multiacidus*
and *Rikenella microfusus*.

	B. capillosus	*M. multiacidus*	*R. microfusus*
Major end-products from PYG[a]	sa (lfp)	LSA (f)	ASp (lf)
Metabolism[b]	NF	F	WF
Dehydrogenases [c] present:-			
MDH	−	+	+
GDH	+[e]	−	−
G6PDH	−	−	−
6PGDH	−	−	−
Major long-chain fatty acid(s)	$C_{14:0}$ $C_{16:0}$	$C_{16:1}$	iso-$C_{15:0}$
Mol % G+C	60	56 − 58	60 − 61

[a] Capital letters refer to major acids; small letters refer to minor
components; letters in parentheses refer to acids which may be
produced; a, acetic; b, butyric; f, formic; l, lactic;
p, propionic; s, succinic.
[b] F, fermentative; NF, non-fermentative; WF, weakly fermentative.
[c] MDH, malate dehydrogenase; GDH, glutamate dehydrogenase;
G6PDH, glucose-6-phoshate dehydrogenase; 6PGDH, 6-phosphogluconate
dehydrogenase.
[e] NADP dependant (Shah and Collins unpublished).

warrant new genera. Biochemical and chemical characteristics of value in the differentiation of these non-
fermentative species and other low mol% G+C containing
taxa are given in Table 3.

Table 3. Biochemical and chemical characteristics useful in the differentiation of non- or weakly fermentative species and other low mol% G+C containing taxa.

	1	2	3	4	5	6
Major end products from PYG[a]	a	B,A,iV	S,A	L,a	A,P,L	A,L(f)
Metabolism[b]	NF	NF	NF	WF	F	F
Dehydrogenase present[c]						
MDH	–	–	ND[d]	–	+	–
GDH	+	–	ND	–	–	–
G6PDH	–	–	ND	+	+	–
6PGH	–	+	ND	–	+	–
Major long-chain fatty acids[e]	$C_{16:0}$ $C_{18:1}$	iso-$C_{15:0}$	$C_{18:1}$	$C_{18:1}$ $C_{18:0}$	$C_{15:0}$	$C_{16:0}$ $C_{18:1}$
Menaquinones produced	ND	ND	ND	–	–	–
Mol% G+C	37	28	28–30	34	32–35	32–30

1. *B. coagulans*; 2. *B. praecutus*; 3. *B. ureolyticus*; 4. *Anaerorhabdus furcosus*; 5. *Megamonas hypermegas*; 6. *Sebaldella termiditis*
[a] Data from Holdeman et al., 1984; iV, isovaleric acid.
[b] NF,non-fermentative; WF,weakly fermentative; F,fermentative
[c] MDH, malate dehydrogenase; GDH, glutamate dehydrogenase; G6PDH, glucose-6-phosphate dehydrogenase; 6PGDH,6-phosphogluconate dehydrogenase
[d] ND,not determined
[e] $C_{15:0}$, pentadecanoic acid; $C_{16:0}$, hexadecanoic acid; $C_{18:0}$, octadecanoic acid; $C_{18:1}$, octadecanoic acid; iso–$C_{15:0}$, 13-methyltetradecanoic acid.

The asaccharolytic pigmented species such as
B. asaccharolyticus, *B. gingivalis* and *B. endodontalis*
possess a mol% G+C range (*ca.* 44–54) which overlaps with
that of true bacteroides (as defined in this chapter)

although they are phenotypically quite distinct from the latter. These species form a biochemically and physiologically homogeneous group which are worthy of separate generic status. Biochemical and chemical properties common to members of this group and which distinguish these from true bacteroides include:

a) production of major amounts of butyric acid (in combination with other acids) as end products of metabolism;

b) are non-fermentative;

c) possess MDH and GDH but lack G6PDH and 6PGDH;

d) produce major amounts of *iso*-methyl branched long-chain fatty acids (with 13-methyltetradecanoic acid predominating).

A variety of other species (eg. *B.macacae*, *B.praeacutus*, *B. levii*) share some, but not all, of the above characteristics. *B.levii* resembles the asaccharolytic pigmented group in producing protohaemin, major amounts of butyric acid (in combination with acetic and other acids) and in possessing a similar dehydrogenase pattern (Shah & Collins 1983, table 1). The DNA base composition of 45-48 mol% G+C reinforces this relatedness. *B. levii*, however, differs in fermenting a few sugars weakly(4). *B.praeacutus* also resembles the asaccharolytic pigmented group in being non-fermentative, producing major levels of butyric acid (in combination with acetic, *iso*-valeric and other acids) and in possessing mainly *iso*-methyl branched long-chain fatty acids with 13-methyltetradecanoic acid predominating (Collins & Shah, unpublished results). The production of an NAD-dependent 6PGDH by *B. praeacutus* together with the absence of MDH and GDH however does not support this relationship (Shah & Collins, 1983). The presence of a significantly lower DNA base composition (i.e. 28 mol% G+C for *B. praeacutus* compared with 44 to 54 mol% G+C for

the asaccharolytic-pigmented group) further emphasises
this difference and indicates *B. praeacutus* warrants a
separate genus. *B. macacae* resembles the asaccharolytic
pigmented group in producing protohaemin although the
production major amounts of propionic and succinic acids
(in combination with small amounts of butyric and other
acids) by the former serves to distinguish these taxa.
Further studies are necessary to clarify the true taxonomic position of *B. macacae*. The taxonomic position of
B. putridinis is also equivocal. *B. putridinis* is similar
to the non-fermentative pigmented group in containing
predominantly *iso*-methyl branched long chain fatty acids
(Collins & Shah, unpublished results). However, it
differs from the latter in producing propionic, succinic
and isovaleric acids as the major end products of metabolism. *B. gracilis*, although asaccharolytic, differs from
the non-fermentative pigmented group in producing succinic
acid as the major end product of metabolism. *B. gracilis*
also differs from the above in producing predominantly
straight-chain saturated and unsaturated long-chain fatty
acids (Collins & Fernandez, unpublished results) and
thermoplasmaquinone (methyl-menaquinone) (1). These data,
together with a mol% G+C value of *ca.* 44 - 46, indicate
that *B.gracilis* should be reclassified in the genus
Wolinella.

B. *melaninogenicus* and related species and the oral
bacteroides (excluding the asaccharolytic species) have
many features in common and may form the basis of a third
major grouping (table 1). Members of this group generally
produce major amounts of acetic and succinic acids (in
combination with other acids) and possess a mol% G+C range
(*ca.* 40-50) which overlaps with those of true bacteroides.

The melaninogenicus/oral group, however, differs from
B. fragilis and related species in lacking the pentose
phosphate pathway enzymes G6PDH and 6PGDH. Further
studies are necessary to establish the homogeneity of this
group.

Biochemical and chemical data indicate that the rumen
species *B. amylophilus* and *B. succinogenes* are unrelated
to *B. fragilis* and related species and should be excluded
from the genus. 16S-rRNA oligonucleotide cataloguing
studies (5) indicate *B. amylophilus* belongs to the phylogenetic unit defined by the purple photosynthetic bacteria
whereas *B. succinogenes* is unrelated to any presently
defined eubacterial 'phyla'.

In Bergey's Manual of Systematic Bacteriology the
genus *Bacteroides* is poorly defined and contains a heterogeneous assortment of obligately anaerobic, Gram-negative,
non-sporeforming rod-shaped bacteria (4). In this article
we have attempted to highlight this unacceptable taxonomic
heterogeneity and have suggested the genus be restricted
to the '*B.fragilis* group' of organisms. The proposed
revision is supported by a wealth of biochemical, physiological and chemical data, and would result in a taxonomically relatively homogeneous genus. Phenotypic data
also indicate that of the 30 or so remaining 'bacteroides'
species, many could be accommodated in the malaninogenicus
/oral and non-fermentative pigmented groups which are
worthy of separate generic status.

References

1   Collins, M.D. & Fernandez, F. 1985. Co-occurence of
     menaquinone-6 and thermoplasmaquinone-6 in *Bacteroides*
     gracilis. FEMS Microbiol. Lett. 26: 181-184.

2   Collins, M.D. and Shah, H.N.   1986.   Reclassification
     of *Bacteroides termitidis* Sebald (Holdeman and Moore)
     in a new genus *Sebaldella*, as *Sebaldella termitidis*
     comb. nov.   Int. J. Syst. Bacterol.   In press.

3   Collins, M.D., Shah, H.N. and Mitsuoka, T.   1985.
     Reclassification of *Bacteroides microfuses* (Kaneuchi
     and Mitsuoka) in a new genus *Rikenella*, as *Rikenella*
     microfuses comb. nov.
     System. Appl. Microbiol. 6: 79-81.

4   Holdeman, L.V., Kelly, R.W. and Moore, W.E.C.   1984.
     Genus *Bacteroides*. Bergey's Manual of Systematic
     Bacteriology Vol. 1.   N.R. Kreig and J.G. Holt, (eds.)
     pp. 604-631.   Baltimore.   Williams and Wilkins.

5   Paster, B.J., Ludwig, W., Weisburg, W.G.,
     Stackebrandt, E., Hespell, R.B., Hahn, C.M.,
     Reichenbach, H., Stetter, K.O. and Woese, C.R.   1985.
     A phylogenetic grouping of the *Bacteroides*,
     cytophagasm and certain flavobacteria.
     System. Appl. Microbiol. 6: 34-42.

6   Shah, H.N. and Collins, M.D. 1982.   Reclassification
     of *Bacteroides hypermegas* (Harrisonand Hansen) in a
     new genus *Megamonas*, as *Megamonas hypermegas* comb.
     nov. Zbl. Bakt. Hyg., 1. Abt. Orig. C3: 394-398.

7   Shah, H.N. and Collins, M.D.   1982.   Reclassification
     of *Bacteroides multiacidus* (Mitsuoka, Terada, Watanabe
     and Uchida) in a new genus *Mitsuokella*, as *Mitsuokella*
     multiacidus comb. nov.
     Zbl. Bakt. Hyg., 1. Abt. Orig. C3: 491-494.

8   Shah, H.N. and Collins, M.D.   1985.   Genus
     Bacteroides: a chemotaxonomical perspective.
     J. Appl. Bacteriol. 55: 403-416.

9   Shah, H.N. and Collins, M.D. 1986.   Reclassification
     of *Bacteroides furcosus* Veillon and Zuber (Hauduroy,
     Ehringer, Urbain, Guillot and Magron) in a new genus
     Anaerorhabdus, as *Anaerorhabdus furcosus* comb. nov.
     System Appl. Microbiol.   In press.

10   Shah, H.N., Kroppenstedt, R.M. and Collins, M.D.
     1983.   Chemical studies as a guide to the
     classification of *Bacteroides hypermegas* and
     Bacteroides multiacidus.
     J. Appl. Bacteriol. 55:   151-158.

CHAPTER 23

THE TAXONOMY OF THE ASACCHAROLYTIC ANAEROBIC GRAM-POSITIVE COCCI

*Taylor E. & Phillips I.

Department of Medical Microbiology, St. Thomas' Hospital, London, SE1.
* Merck, Sharp & Dohme, Hertford Road,Hoddesdon, Herts., UK.

Contents

Abstract

Introduction

      Conventional Classification

      Identification

Recent Chemotaxonomic studies

      Cell-wall structure

      Protein electrophoresis

      Nucleic acids

References

ABSTRACT

The taxonomy of the Peptococcacae is poorly understood and in recent years has undergone much amendment. In 1980, there were seven recognised species within the genus *Peptococcus* and four within the genus *Peptostreptococcus*. Today, there is only one *Peptococcus* species – the type species *P. niger*, and seven *Peptostreptococcus* species – *Ps.micros*, *Ps.magnus*, *Ps.productus*, *Ps.asaccharolyticus*, *Ps. prevotii*, *Ps. indolicus* and *Ps. anaerobius*.

Recent changes in the taxonomic status of the Peptococaceae have largely been based on new chemotaxonomic techniques, such as DNA-base ratios and nucleic acid hybridisation studies. Simple and reliable methods for the differentation and taxonomy of these organisms have not yet been described.

INTRODUCTION

Improvements in anaerobic technology and an increased awareness of the role that anaerobes play in clinical infection have led to the isolation of hitherto unfamiliar organisms in clinical microbiology laboratories. This has been particularly true of the anaerobic Gram-positive cocci, which, together with the bacteroides, are the most commonly isolated anaerobes in human infection (6,8).

Unfortunately, the increased clinical interest in anaerobic Gram-positive cocci has been matched by an even greater increase in the confusion concerning their taxonomy, classification and identifciation. Most species appear assacharolytic, so that carbohydrate fermentation tests, the back-bone of classical taxonomic systems, are useless and few other species-specific characteristics have been reported.

The Conventional Classification. Knowledge of the existence of anaerobic cocci dates from the work of Veillon in 1893, who isolated an anaerobic coccus, which he named *Micrococcus foetidus* from a casé of Bartholinitis. During the first half of the 20th century, various attempts were made to classify these organisms, and in 1924, Prevot made his first attempts at a classification system. His research continued for the next quarter of a century, culminating in the publication of his "Manuel de classification et de determination des bacteries anaerobies" in 1948/9. This system, based entirely on morphological and biochemical characteristics, gained widespread approval, and has formed the basis of most subsequent attempts to classify the Peptococcaceae.

However, a very different classification system was developed by Hare in London at about the same time. This classification system has been largely ignored outside the United Kingdom, but merits attention as much of the more recent research on these organisms has shown many of Hare's ideas to be correct, and because the National Type Culture Collection of anaerobic cocci are identified by their Hare Group only. Hare was clearly critical of Prevot's work and found that the majority of his strains could not be identified by Prevot's criteria. He argued that the metabolic requirements of the anaerobic cocci were so complex that, unless strictly standardised media were used, fermentation tests became meaningless (4). His experiments showed that the results of fermentation tests were particularly affected by varying concentrations of fatty acids or sulphur compounds in the growth medium.

His observation, if correct, would imply the incorrect description of 'new species', and as *Ps.anaerobius* now has the dubious honour of no less than nine synonyms (3), it would appear that this may well have been the case.

More recent research into the taxonomy of these organisms has been performed firstly, by Louis D. Smith, and later, by Holdeman, Cato and Moore at the Virginia Polytechnic Institute. The Anaerobe Laboratory Manual, published by this group of workers, has become the internationally recognised reference work for the identification and classification of anaerobic bacteria. The fourth edition of this manual was brought out in 1977 and lists six species of peptococci and four species of peptostreptococci, characterised by their volatile fatty acid profile and reactions in carbohydrate fermentation tests (5). This listing, with the exception of the exclusion of *Peptococcus glycinophilus*, exactly matches that published in the Approved Lists of Bacterial Names by Skerman, McGowan and Sneath (11), produced to clarify the taxonomic status of the almost infinite number of species named in earlier publications. In addition, the Approved List refers almost exclusively to the VPI Manual for the species description of the recognised Peptococcaceae. Thus, in practice, the characteristics used for the taxonomy of these organisms reflect those available for their routine identification.

Identification. As can be seen in Table 1, these organisms are generally asaccharolytic, and only *Ps.productus* can be identified by positive reactions in carbohydrate fermentation tests. It is of interest that both the type species of the genus *Peptococcus* - *P.niger*, and the type species of the genus *Peptostreptococcus* -

Table 1. Identification of the anaerobic Gram Positive cocci.

	1	2	3	4	5	6	7	8
Carbohydrate fermentation tests	– or weak	–	–	–	–	–	–	+
Indole	–	–	+	+	–	–	–	–
Nitrate	–w	–	–	–	–	–	–	–
Coagulase	–	–	–	+	–	–	–	–
Cell size						>0.6mm	<0.6mm	
VFA production	A,p, ib,b iv,IC	A,p, ib,b, iv,C	A,p, B	A,p, B	A,p, B	A	A	A

1. *Ps. anaerobius*, 2. *P. niger*, 3. *Ps. asaccharolyticus*,
4. *Ps. indolicus*, 5. *Ps. prevotii*, 6. *Ps. magnus*, 7. *Ps. micros*
8. *Ps. productus*.

Ps. anaerobius have characteristic volatile fatty acid (VFA) profiles that are quite different from those of the remaining species.   These can be allocated to one of two groups according to whether butyrate is or is not produced.

For the most part, identification is dependant on one or occasionally two positive tests. *Ps. anaaerobius* is identified by its characteristic VFA pattern, the butyrate-producing cocci are speciated on the basis of indole and coagulase production, and *Ps. magnus* is separated from *Ps. micros* on the basis of size alone. It is not surprising, therefore that most clinical microbiologists have little confidence in their ability to identify these organisms.

Antibiotic sensitivity testing has been suggested as a means of providing a rapid provisional identification of the anaerobic Gram-positive cocci. Sutter and her colleagues (14) reported that vancomycin sensitivity distinguished the Gram-negative from the Gram-positive and

Watt & Jack (15) suggested that metronidazole sensitivity
could be used to differentiate the micro-aerophilic from
the 'true' anaerobe. In addition, Wren and his co-workers
(18) suggested that novobiocin sensitivity could be used
to differentiate members of the genus *Peptococcus* (as it
then stood) from the *Peptostreptococci*. Wren reported
that the peptostreptococci were sensitive to novobiocin,
but later work has shown that the species *Ps. micros* is
resistant (Taylor, unpublished observations). Finally,
sodium polyanethanol sulphonate (SPS) sensitivity has been
suggested for the presumptive identification of

Table 2. Presumptive rapid identification of anaerobic
cocci by disc sensitivity tests.

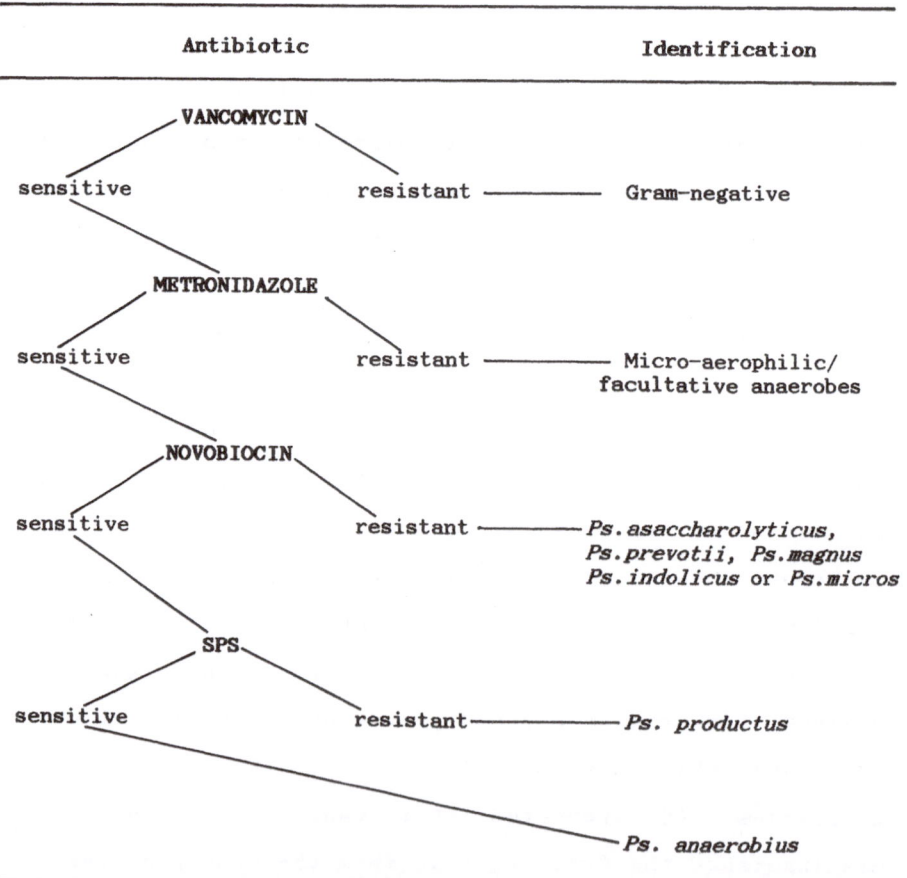

Ps. anaerobius (17). An outlined suggested scheme for the provisional identification of the anaerobic Gram-positive cocci based on disc sensitivity testing is shown in Table 2.

RECENT CHEMOTAXONOMIC STUDIES

In the last decade, there have been several attempts to use new chemotaxonomic techniques to re-examine the anaerobic cocci.

Examination of the cell-wall structure. It has been suggested that the peptidoglycan stucture of the cell-wall is species-specific (10). Weiss (18) determined the cell wall structure of representatives of most of the recognised species within the genera *Peptococcus* and *Peptostreptococcus*, together with those of the Hare Group organisms. He used this technique to group *Ps. anaerobius* with *P. niger*, and to group *Ps. magnus* with Hare Group IV and two recognised synonyms of *Ps. magnus* – *Ps. variabilis* and *Peptococcus anaerobius*. He also concluded from this work that there was some heterogeneity within the butyrate -producing cocci and that some strains, identified as *Ps.prevotii* or *Ps. asaccharolyticus* by conventional tests, had the same cell- wall structure.

Recently, Schleifer's group have reported on the diversity of peptidoglycan structure of some closely related anaerobic cocci, as judged by nucleic acid homology studies (7). It would appear that, although determination of the cell-wall structure is a valuable taxonomic tool for most Gram-positive species, care must be taken in deducing the relationship of the anaerobic Gram-positive cocci solely on the basis of peptidoglycan structure.

Whole-cell protein electrophoresis. Cato and her colleagues (1) used whole-cell protein electrophoresis to

266

demonstrate heterogeneity within the species *Ps. magnus*, suggesting that the species *Ps. variabilis* should be re-instated. At the same time, Cato also reported that the results of protein electrophoresis supported her belief that *P. glycinophilus* was a synonym of *Ps. micros*. More recently, Taylor and co-workers (14) have used whole-cell protein electrophoresis to demonstrate heterogeneity within the species *Ps. asaccharolyticus* and to illustrate that the indole test is unreliable for the speciation of the butyrate- producing cocci. In this study whole-cell protein electrophoresis also showed heterogeneity within the species *Ps.magnus* and the homogeneity of the species *Ps. anaerobius* and *Ps. micros*. These workers also con-cluded that Hare Group IV is synonymous with *Ps. magnus* and that Hare Group IX is synonymous with the species *Ps. micros*, supporting the observations of Weiss (17).

Table 3. Published results on DNA-base ratios (2)

SPECIES	G + C %
P.niger	50-51
Ps.anaerobius	33-35
Ps.asaccharolyticus	32-38
Ps.indolicus	32-34
Ps.magnus	32-34
Ps.prevotii	32-34
Ps.micros	27-29
Ps.productus	44-45

Nucleic acid Studies. Table 3 lists the published DNA-base ratios of the recognised species. *P. niger* has a high

G+C% of 50-51%, which is clearly different from that of
the other peptococci. There is marked heterogeneity within
the genus *Peptostreptococcus*, with a range in DNA-base
ratios of 28-45%. Ezaki and his colleagues (2) used this
difference in DNA-base ratios to support their transfer of
four species - *P.asaccharolyticus*, *P.prevotii*, *P.indolicus*
and *P.magnus* - to the genus *Peptostreptococcus*. Ezaki and
his colleagues also performed DNA-homology studies on the
Peptococcaceae and found that there was 23-38% homology
between these species and *Ps. anaerobius* but negligible
homology with *P. niger*, the type species of the genus
Peptococcus. In addition, Ezaki reported on marked
heterogeneity within the species *Ps. prevotii*, finding
that the DNA-DNA homology between the type strain and
clinical isolates ranged from 0-75%. He also concluded
that there were two distinct groups within the species
Ps.asaccharolyticus.

A later study by Huss and his colleagues (7) confirmed
heterogeneity among the butyrate-producing cocci, but did
not support the transfer of *P.asaccharolyticus*, *P.prevotii*,
P.magnus and *P.indolicus* to the genus Peptostreptococcus.
Instead, these workers found that the type species of this
genus, *Ps. anaerobius*, was more closely related to
Eubacterium tenue and *Clostridium lituseburense* than to
any of the other anaerobic Gram-positive cocci.

As nucleic acid studies are currently recognised as
the definitive tool for microbial taxonomics, it must be
accepted that the classification of the anaerobic Gram-
positive cocci remains in a very unsatisfactory state.
There is mounting evidence that the type species of both
the genus *Peptococcus* and *Peptostreptococcus* were ill-
chosen, and that other species that we consider as members

of either genus are only remotely related to their respective type species.

In addition, we have to accept that many of the currently recognised 'bench tests' for species identification are variable and therefore quite unsuitable for routine use. It is clear that the accurate identification of these very difficult organisms will remain beyond the capabilities of most microbiologists for many years to come. Further detailed taxonomic studies on the Peptococcaceae are eagerly awaited.

References

1   Cato, E.P., Johnson, J.L., Hash, D.E. and Holdeman, L.V. 1983. Synonymy of *Peptococcus glycinophilus* (Cardon and Barker 1946) Douglas 1957 with *Peptostreptococcus micros* (Prevot 1933) Smith 1957 and electrophoretic differentiation of *Peptostreptococcus micros* from *Peptococcus magnus* (Prevot 1933) Holdeman and Moore 1972. Int. J. Syst. Bacteriol. 33: 207-210

2   Ezaki, T., Yamamoto, N., Ninomiya, K., Suzuki, S. and Yabuuchi, E. 1983. Transfer of *Peptococcus* indolicus, Peptococcus asaccharolyticus, Peptococcus prevotii *and* Peptococcus magnus *to the genus* Peptostreptococcus and proposal of *Peptostreptoccus tetradius* sp.nov. Int. J. Syst. Bacteriol. 33: 883-898

3   Finegold, S.F. 1977. Anaerobic bacteria in human disease. Academic Press, New York

4   Hare, R. 1967. The anaerobic cocci. In Recent advances in Medical Microbiology. Waterson A.P. (editor). J & A Churchill Ltd., W.l. p.284-317

5   Holdeman, L.V., Cato, E.P. and Moore, W.E.C. 1977. Anaerobe Laboratory Manual, (4th edition), Viriginia Polytechnic Institute and State University, Blacksburg, Va.,

6   Holland, J.W., Hill, E.O. and Altemeier, W.A. 1976. Numbers and types of anaerobic bacteria isolated from clinical specimens since 1960. J. Clin. Microbiol. 5: 20-25

7   Huss, V.A.R., Festl, H. and Schleifer, K.H. 1984. Nucleic acid hybridisation studies and deoxyribonucleic acid base compositions of anaerobic, Gram-positive cocci. Int. J. Syst. Bacteriol. 34: 95-101

8   Phillips, I. 1981. General review of anaerobic infections. Revue de L'Institut Pasteur de Lyons 14: 243-249

9   Prevot, A.R. 1948. Manuel de classification et de determination des bacteries anaerobies. Paris, Masson.

10 Schleifer, K.H. and Kandler, O. 1972. Peptidoglycan types of bacterial cell walls and their taxonomic implications. Bacteriol. Rev. 36: 407-477

11 Skerman, V.B.D., McGowan, V. and Sneath, P.H.A. 1980. Approved lists of bacterial names. Int. J. Syst. Bacteriol. 30 225-420

12 Sutter, V.L., Vargo, V.L. and Finegold, S.M. 1975. Wadsworth anaerobic bacteriology manual, 2nd ed. University of California, Los Angeles, Extension Division, Los Angeles.

13 Taylor, E.A. 1984. The taxonomy of the
    asaccharolytic anaerobic Gram-positive cocci. PhD
    thesis. University of London.

14 Taylor, E., Jackman, P.J.H. and Phillips, I. Whole-
    cell protein electrophoresis and the taxonomy of the
    asaccharolytic anaerobic Gram-positive cocci (In
    prep.)

15 Watt, B. and Jack, E.P. 1977. What are anaerobic
    cocci? J. Med. Microbiol. 10: 481-468

16 Weiss, N. 1981.   Cell wall structure of anaerobic
    cocci. Rev. Inst. Pasteur Lyon. 14: 53-59

17 Wideman, P.A., Vargo, V.L., Citronbaum, D. and
    Finegold, S.M. 1976. Evaluation of the Sodium
    Polyanethol Sulfonate disk test for the identification
    of *Peptostreptococcus anaerobius*.
    J. Clin. Microbiol. 4: 330-333

18 Wren, M.W.D., Eldon, C.P. and Dakin, G.H. 1977.
    Novobiocin and the differentiation of peptococci and
    peptostreptococci. J. Clin. Path. 30: 620-622

CHAPTER 24

TAXONOMY OF SPIRAL AND CURVED CLOSTRIDIA

R.J. Carman, Elizabeth P. Cato and Tracy D. Wilkins

Department of Anaerobic Microbiology, Virginia Polytechnic
Institute and State University, Blacksburg, Virginia 24061,
USA.

Contents

Abstract

Introduction

Materials and Methods

    Bacterial strains

    Biochemical characterization

    In vivo MIC determinations

    Electrophoresis of soluble
    cellular proteins

    Crossed immunoelectrophoresis

    Toxin assays

Results

    Biochemical characterizations

    In vivo MICs

    Soluble cellular protein
    electrophoretogram

    Crossed immunoelectrophoretograms

    Toxicities

Conclusions

References

272

ABSTRACT

Seventy seven curved and helically coiled, anaerobic bacilli, which were isolated from the intestinal contents of humans, rabbits and chickens, were the subject of this study. Because they were anaerobic, spore forming, Gram positive rods the isolates were identified as clostridia. Those strains which seemed to have a helically coiled cellular conformation were in fact microcolonies of semi-circular cells joined end to end. The strains fell into five groups on the basis of their biochemical characteristics, their susceptibilities to a range of antimicrobial agents, their outer membrane protein and extracellular toxins. Group 1 contained three strains of *Clostridium spiroforme*, including the type strain, isolated from healthy humans who had not been receiving antibiotics. None of these isolates produced a toxin. Although similar in some respects to the members of Groups 2 and 3, they do in fact represent a distinct group. Groups 2 and 3 share some common extracellular antigens. The former consists of three strains of *C.spiroforme* isolated from diarrhoeic humans who had received clindamycin, the latter was made up of 59 strains of *C. spiroforme* from scouring rabbits. All of the rabbit strains, but none of the human isolates, produced a lethal toxin neutralizable with *C. perfringens* iota antitoxin. Group 4 contained six unnamed strains isolated from healthy chickens. None were toxigenic. They differed in most aspects from the *C. spiroforme* strains but did share some properties with

C. cocleatum, the organism represented in group 5. It is not yet clear whether or not group 2 and 3 should be given species status separate from *C. spiroforme*. For the time being, however, we are continuing to refer to them as *C. spiroforme*.

INTRODUCTION

In 1979 Kaneuchi *et al* (7) described four different groupings of curved clostridia, two of which were assigned species status: *C. spiroforme* and *C. cocleatum*. Both these species have been isolated from the intestinal contents of man and other animals. However it was assumed that they were commensals until the causal role of *C. spiroforme* in an acute infectious diarrhoea of rabbits was established. Since the cause and effect relationship was reported, several workers, including ourselves, have questioned the validity of placing the rabbit pathogenic strains with *C. spiroforme*. Three strains of *C. spiroforme* and six *C. cocleatum* isolated from humans with clindamycin – associated diarrhoea, from whom no *C. difficile* could be isolated and whose faecal filtrates contained no neutralizable *C. difficile* cytoxin, futher prompted us to reconsider the taxonomic status of the isolates with which we were working. Using several different approaches 77 strains falling within the scope of Kaneuchi's (1979)(7) definition of helically coiled, sporeforming anaerobes were examined.

MATERIALS AND METHODS

Bacterial strains. The 77 strains studied and their sources are listed in Table 1. All of the strains were originally isolated from faeces or caecal content. Following purification they had been either lyophilized or

Table 1.   Sources and origins of strains

Group	Species	Sources	Origin
1 (3)*	*C. spiroforme*	VPI, USA	Healthy human stool
2 (3)	*C. spiroforme*	VPI, USA	Human clindamycin assoicated diarrhoea
3 (69)	*C. spiroforme*	London, UK Rouen, France St Louis, USA Wilmington, USA	Diarrhoeic rabbit faeces and caeca
4. (6)	Unnamed	Norwich, UK	Healthy chicken faeces
5 (6)	*C. cocleatum*	VPI, USA	Human clindamycin associated diarrhoea

* Numbers in brackets indicate number of strains examined

stored in chopped meat broths at room temperature.   Prior to these studies the organisms were revived by anaerobic culture on freshly prepared rabbit blood agar.   Single colonies were subcultured onto additional blood agar plates to provide appropriate material for the project.

Biochemical characterization.   The techniques used were those described in the VPI Anaerobe Laboratory Manual (6). The tests employed are shown in Table 2.

Minimal inhibitory concentration (MIC) determination. Using the methods of Sutter *et al* (1979) (8) the MIC levels of the several antimicrobial agents (Table 3) were measured.

Electrophoresis of soluble cellular proteins.   The soluble cellular proteins of the different strains grown in brain heart infusion broths (BHI) supplemented with Tween 80 (0.025%) were analysed by polyacrylamide gel electro-phoresis (PAGE).   The methods used have been described by Cato *et al* (1982) (5).

Table 2. Some biochemical reactions of curved clostridia

Test	1	2	3	4	5
Amygdalin	−	a^-	−	a^-	a
Arabinose	−	−	−	$-^a$	−
Cellobiose	−	a	−	a^-	a
Erythritol	−	−	−	−	−
Aesculin pH	−	a	−	a	a^-
Aesculin hydrolysis	−	+	−	+	+
Fructose	w	a	a	a^-	a
Glucose	w	a	a	a	a
Glycogen	−	−	−	−	−
Inositol	−	−	−	−	−
Lactose	w	a^w	a	a^-	a
Maltose	−	−	−	−	−
Mannitol	−	−	a	−	−
Mannose	w	a	a	a	a
Melezitose	−	−	−	−	−
Melibiose	−	−	−	−	−
Raffinose	−	−	a^-	−	$-^a$
Rhamnose	−	−	$-^w$	$-^a$	−
Ribose	−	$-^w$	−	a^-	$-^w$
Salicin	−	a^w	−	a^w	a
Sorbitol	−	−	−	$-^a$	−
Starch pH	−	−	−	a^-	−
Starch hydrolysis	−	−	−	−	−
Sucrose	a	a	a	$-^a$	a
Trehalose	−	−	$-^w$	a^-	−
Xylose	−	−	w^a	$-^a$	−
Gelatin	−	−	−	−	−
Milk	c	c	c	c	c
Meat	−	−	−	−	−
Indole	−	−	−	−	−
Catalase	−	−	−	−	−
Lecithinase	−	−	−	−	−
Lipase	−	−	−	−	−
Haemolysis	−	−	−	−	−
Pectin	ND	−	−	−	ND

Legend of symbols:-
    + = positive reaction for almost all strains
    − = negative reaction for almost all stains
    a = strong acid, pH 5.5 or below
    c = curd
    w = weak acid, pH 5.5 to 6.0
    Supersrcipts = reactions of occasional strains
    ND = Not done

<u>Crossed immunoelectrophoresis</u>.   Using the general crossed
immunoelectrophoresis methods reported in Axelson *et al*
(1973) (1),   ten fold concentrates of culture supernatants
were examined. Bacteria were grown for 48h at 37°C in BHI
supplemented with proteose peptone (1%),   glucose (1%) and

divalant cations (5microM).   Antigen samples (15 microlitre) were run against goat antiserum to *C.spiroforme* NCTC 11493. The resultant crossed patterns gave us information on both iota   toxin   production   and   on   the   degree   of   cross reactivity between the collection of strains and the known rabbit pathogen.

Toxin assays.   Bacteria were grown in BHI peptone glucose divalant   cation   medium   (see above)   for   48h   at   37°C. Sterile   culture filtrates were injected intraperitoneally into mice (0.5 ml/mouse;   2 mice per   sample).   Organisms were deemed to be toxic if both mice died within 48 hours.

Table   3.   Minimal inhibitory concentrations (MIC) of antimicrobial agents to curved clostridia

| Agent | Range of MIC/ microgrammes per ml^{-1} | | |
	Group 2	Group 3	Group 4
Bacitracin	0.25	4 – > 8	0.25 – 0.5
Cefoxitin	0.016	2 – 4	0.016 – 0.5
Chloramphenicol	0.063	0.125 – 0.25	0.063 – 0.25
Erythromycin	0.125 – >8	0.25 – >8	0.063
Kanamycin	4 – >8	4 – >8	4 – >8
Lincomycin	0.063 – >8	0.5 – >8	0.063 – 0.25
Mefoxin	0.016 – 4	0.125 – >8	0.125 – >8
Naladixic Acid	>8	>8	>8
Penicillin G	0.008 – 0.016	<0.004 – 0.125	<0.004 – 0.125
Rifampicin	0.008	>8	0.008
Tetracycline	0.016 – 0.063	0.25 – >8	0.063
Vancomycin	0.031	2 – >8	0.031

RESULTS

Biochemical   characterization.   Based   upon   the   data gathered   during these studies,   five groups of   organisms were   established.   Their biochemical reactions are given by group in Table 2.

Minimal inhibitory concentrations.   The *in vitro* response of   the   different   strains to a   range   of   antimicrobial agents   was measured on three occasions.   The results   are shown in Table 3.

Soluble cellular protein electrophoresis. The electro-
phoretograms showed that there was considerable homogeneity when comparisons were made between groups 2 and 3
(Table 1) and, to a lesser extent, between groups 4 and 5.

Crossed immunoelectrophoresis. Crossed immunoelectrophoresis of strains against antiserum to the known toxigenic pathogen *C.spiroforme* NCTC 11493, showed that only
the rabbit strains were capable of producing sufficient
iota toxin for it to be detected using this technique.
The antigenic relatedness of groups 2 and 3, initially
shown using PAGE, was further established. Up to twenty
common precipitin arcs were apparant. No isolates from
groups other than 2 and 3 contained antigens precipitated
by this antiserum.

Toxin assays. All 77 strains were tested for toxin
production in a variety of media. Al those isolates from
diarrhoeic rabbits produced a mouse lethal toxin which was
neutralizable with iota antitoxins. No other strains
could be shown to be toxigenic *in vitro*.

5. CONCLUSIONS

Seventy seven strains of similarly shaped intestinal
clostridia were examined. superficially they fell into 3
groups; *C. spiroforme, C. cocleatum* and an unnamed group.
Our researches have convinced us that this impression is
too simple. Whilst we still feel that *C. cocleatum* is a
valid grouping, as is the collection under one heading of
the avian isolates, *C. spiroforme* may well consist of
three distinct species. The first would include the type
strain and those isolates from healthy human faeces. The
second would be made up of those strains from diarrhoeic

humans following treatment with antibiotics. The third and final group includes those iota toxigenic isolates from cases of spontaneous and antibiotic assoiated diarrhoea of rabbits.

Our reasons for making these divisions are the major differences in MICs, toxin production, biochemical reactions, antigenic profiles and apparant pathogenicity between the three groups currently gathered under the heading, *C. spiroforme*. However further tests to validate these divisions are necessary. Such tests include measurement of G+C% ratios and DNA:DNA hybridisation. Meanwhile we are continuing to include the pathogenic rabbit strains and the potentially pathogenic human strains in *C.spiroforme*.

References

1   Axelsen, N.H., Kroll, J. and Weeke, B. (eds.) 1973.   A
     manual of quantitative immunoelectrophoresis.   Methods
     and applications.   Scand. J. Immun. 2 (S1): 1-169.

2   Borriello, S.P. and Carman, R.J. 1983.   Association of
     iota-like toxin and *Clostridium spiroforme* with both
     spontaneous and antibiotic- associated diarrhea and
     colitis in rabbits.   J. Clin. Microbiol. 17: 414-18.

3   Carman, R.J. and Borriello, S.P. 1982a. Observation on
     an association between *Clostridium spiroforme* and
     Clostridium.   Journal Chemother. Antibiot. 2: 143-44.

4   Carman, R.J., and Borriello, S.P. 1982b.   *Clostridium
     spiroforme* isolated from rabbbits with diarrhoea.
     Vet. Rec. 111: 461-62.

5   Cato, E.P., Hash, D.E., Holderman, L.V. *et al.* 1982.
     Electrophoretic study of *Clostridium* species.
     J. Clin. Microbiol. 15: 688-702.

6   Holdeman, L.V., Cato, E.P. and Moore, W.E.C. (eds.).
     1977.   Anaerobe laboratory manual, 4th ed. Virginia
     Polytechnic Institute and State University,
     Blacksburg, Va.

7   Kaneuchi, C. Miyazato, T., Shinjo, T., *et al.* 1979.
     Taxonomic study of helically coiled, sporeforming
     anaerobes isolated from the intestines of humans and
     other animals: *Clostridium* colcleatum *sp. nov. and
     Clostridium spiroforme* sp. nov.
     Int. J. Syst. Bacteriol. 29: 1-12.

8   Sutter, V.L., Barry, A.L., Wilkins, T.D. *et al* 1979.
     Collaborative evaluation of a proposed reference
     dilution method of susceptibility testing of anaerobic
     bacteria.   Antimicrob. Agents Chemother: 16: 495-502.

ABSTRACTS OF POSTERS PRESENTED AT THE 4th ADG BIENNIAL
SYMPOSIUM, CAMBRIDGE, 1985.

INDEX

1. The PBPs of *Bacteroides thetaiotaomicron* and their
    role in the susceptibility to beta-lactamase
    antibiotics. L.J.V. Piddock and R. Wise.

2. Susceptibility of *Bacteroides* species to cefotetan
    and four other antimicrobial angents. M. Wilks and
    Soad Tabaqchali.

3. NCTC 11870: A new control organism for susceptibility
    testing of anaerobes. J.R. Edwards and P.J. Turner.

4. Biochemical and chemical studies on some poorly
    characterised, non-fermentative *Bacteroides* species.
    H.N. Shah and M.D. Collins.

5. Inhibition of *Bacteroides vulgatus* and zymosan of the
    killing of *Escherichia coli* by polymorphonuclear
    leukocytes. W.A.C. Vel, F. Namavar, A.M.J.J. Verweij,
    A.N.B. Pubben and D.M. MacLaren.

6. The use of fast protein liquid chromatography for the
    identification of anaerobic bacteria.
    S.P. Borriello, P.J. Reed and Fiona E. Barclay.

7. Microtube plate procedure for biochemical
    characterization and antimicrobial susceptibility
    testing of anaerobic bacteria. S.D. Allen,
    J.A. Siders, N.B. O'Bryan, and E.H. Gerlach.

8. Faecal anaerobe flora and faecal vitamin K
    concentrations in response to diet and antimicrobial
    agents: Investigations with moxalactam, cefoperazone
    and clindamycin. S.D. Allen, J.A. Siders,
    C.G. Kindberg, P.M. Allison, N.U. Bang, M.D. Cromer,
    N.B. O'Bryan, G.L. Brier, and J.H. Suttie.

9. Composition of bacterial flora in ilial reservoir
    patients. M.D. Holdom, M.J. Hill, R.L. Moskowitz and
    R.J. Nicholls.

10. Food intolerance and microbial populations in the
    human colon. Hazel K. Bradley, Catherine E. Bayliss,
    G.M. Wyatt, Anne F. Smith, Virginia A. Jones and
    J.O. Hunter.

11. Impact of different antimicrobial agents on the
    anaerobic oropharyngeal and intestinal microflora.
    C.E. Nord and A. Heimdahl.

12. Colonization resistance to *Clostridium difficile:*
    evaluation of volatile fatty acid concentration in
    caecal contents from different types of animals.
    W.J. Su, M.J. Waechter, M. Dolegeal. P. Bourlioux and
    G. Mahuzier.

13. Identification of *Clostridium difficile* using the API
    Zym system. P.N. Levett.

14. An immunochemical fingerprinting method for
    Clostridium difficile. Jacqueline Sharp and
    I.R. Poxton.

15. Iota toxin produced by both *clostridium spiroforme*
    and *Clostridium perfringens* Type E is a synergistic
    combination of two proteins. R.J. Carman, B.G. Stiles,
    and T.D. Wilkins.

16. The use of *Bacteroides fragilis* group as indicators
    of sewage pollution of environmental waters.
    R.J. Carman.

17. Anaerobe holding chamber. J.D. Brown and Wendy J. Smith.

18. Isolation of anaerobes in the routine laboratory.
    K.W. Bennett and B.I. Duerden.

19. The possible role of anaerobes in methylmalonic
    aciduria, an inherited metabolic disease.
    S.P. Borriello, P.J. Reed, M. Bain, M. Jones,
    M.N. Tracey, T.E. Stacey and R.A. Chalmers.

20. Influence of sulphatase-producing intestinal bacteria
    on the metabolism of bile salts and steroid hormones.
    H. Eyssen, J. van Eldere and J. Robban.

21. Food additive metabolism by intestinal bacteria in
    man. P. Geraldine S. Cook.

22. Maintenance in continuous culture of the gastric
    microflora of a hypochlorhydric patient.
    T.M. Coutts, A.J. Alldrick, I.R. Rowland, J.M. Dolby
    and S.P. Borriello.

23. A chemostat model for formation of bacterial films on
    acrylic tiles. D.J. Bradshaw, A.B. Dowsett and
    C.W. Keevil.

24. Characterization of colonial varaints on *Bacteroides
    gingivalis* W50 with an altered virulence for mice.
    Ailsa S. McKee, Ann S. McDermid, A.B. Dowsett,
    A. Baskerville and P.D. Marsh.

25. The growth of *Actinomyces naeslundii* in the dental
    plaque of monkeys *(Macaca fascicularis).*
    D. Beighton and H. Hayday.

26. Attaching spirochaetes in the pig colon. R.J. Lysons,
    A.P.Bland and M.R. Burrows .

27. Plasmids in steroid nuclear dehydrogenating
    clostridia. Daphne E. Thompson, B.S. Drasar and
    A.R. Cook.

ABSTRACT   1

THE PBPs OF *BACTEROIDES THETAIOTAOMICRON* AND THEIR ROLE IN THE SUSCEPTIBILITY TO BETA-LACTAM ANTIBIOTICS.

L.J.V. Piddock and R. Wise

Microbiology Department, Dudley Road Hospital, Birmingham, U.K.

Bacteroides thetaiotaomicron has been shown to be less susceptible to Beta-lactam antibiotics than other species of the same genus. Resistance to Beta-lactam antibiotics by members of the genus *Bacteroides* has been attributed to potent Beta-lactamases, however newer Beta-lactamase stable compounds show little improvement in efficacy against *B. thetaiotaomicron*; to obtain a further understanding of this species and its susceptibility to Beta-lactams, the PBPs and their affinity to 35 Beta-lactam compounds were examined. Using SDS-polyacrylamide electrophoresis four PBPs were resolved from envelopes of *B. thetaiotaomicron* (Figure) which are all fully saturated by 40 mcg/ml^{-1} [^{14}C] benzylpenicillin. The PBP competition data (Table) demonstrates that most compounds bind primarily to PBP 2, then PBP 1, which is correlated with the morphological response of filamentation, then sphaeroplasting and lysis. N-F thienamycin and methicillin bound to PBP 3 primarily causing rounding of cells and bulging filaments. By comparing the data from this study with the PBP data for *Escherichia coli*, it is proposed that the PBPs from *B. thetaiotaomicron* have the following functions: PBP 1 is an enzyme involved in cell elongation, PBP 2 is an enzyme involved in septum formation and PBP 3 is an enzyme involved in the maintenance of cell shape. Several compounds (aztreonam, cefamandole, cefaclor) had PBP I$_{50}$ well below the MIC which may indicate the presence of a penetration barrier (due to periplasmic Beta-lactamase or

Table. Competition of Beta-lactam antibiotics for the PBPs of envelope preparations of *Bacteroides thetaiotaomicron*.

Antibiotic	Agar dilution MIC 10^4	10^6	PBP ID$_{50}$ (mcg/ml^{-1}) 1a	1b	2	3	4	Morphological response
Amoxycillin	32	64	8	8	8	>1024	8	(F) + S
Methicillin	32	64	32	32	<8	16	64	BF
Penicillin G	16	16	8	8	8	>1024	>1024	F + S
Ticarcillin	32	64	<8	<8	8	64	512	F
Temocillin	64	128	1024	1024	256	>1024	>1024	F
Cephalexin	8	16	>256	>256	2	32	>256	F
Cefamandole	32	64	64	64	>256	16	128	BF
Cefoxitin	16	16	4	4	16	64	32	S (+ L)
Cefuroxime	16	32	128	128	32	>512	128	F
Cefaclor	128	128	64	64	<16	16	64	F + S
Cefsulodin	128	>128	128	128	128	256	>256	(F) + S
Ceftazidime	8	8	16	16	>256	8	>256	S
Aztreonam	128	>128	512	512	32	512	512	F
N-F-thienamycin	0.5	0.5	1	1	0.5	0.06	>32	BF + R
Moxalactam	4	4	8	8	8	>1024	>1024	F + L

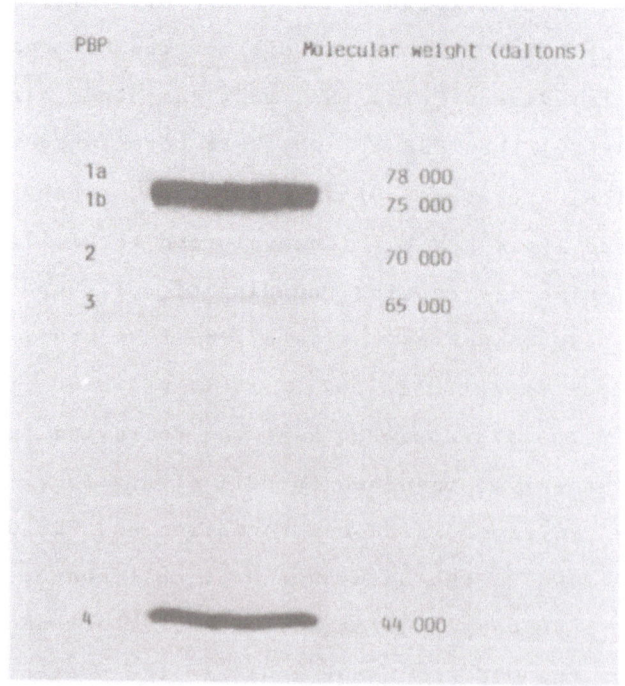

PBP   Molecular weight (daltons)

1a   78 000
1b   75 000

2   70 000

3   65 000

4   44 000

outer membrane or a combination of both phenomena).
Several compounds (temocillin, cefuroxime, methicillin,
cefsulodin) had ID_{50} at relatively high concentrations
correlating with high MIC, indicating that low affinity of
the PBPs for these compounds may cause low susceptibility.

ABSTRACT 2

SUSCEPTIBILITY OF *BACTEROIDES* SPECIES TO CEFOTETAN AND FOUR OTHER ANTIMICROBIAL AGENTS.

M. Wilks and S. Tabaqchali

Department of Medical Microbiology, St. Bartholomew's
Hospital Medical College, West Smithfield, London, UK.

Cefotetan is a new long acting injectable cephamycin
with a broad antimicrobial spectrum. The activity of
cefotetan was determined against 206 strains of
Bacteroides spp. by means of an agar dilution test, and
compared with that of cefoxitin, cefotaxime, clindamycin
and metronidazole.

Inocula were prepared by picking isolated colonies
into Wilkins-Chalgren broth supplemented with 1% inacti-
vated horse serum (2). The broth was diluted to provide
10^4 cfu when applied to the surface of the test medium,
Wilkins-Chalgren agar plus 7% defibrinated horse- blood,
with a Denley multipoint inoculator.

The cephalosporins showed considerable variation in
their action against different species. Against *B.fragilis*
(46 strains), cefotetan and cefoxitin gave very similar
results with 89% and 91% of strains inhibited at 16 mg/l
respectively. Cefotaxime was less active with only 28% of
strains inhibited at 16mg/l and an MIC_{90} of 128mg/l.

The other less pathogenic members of the *B. fragilis* group were more resistant with MIC90s of 128, 64 and >128mg/l respectively. Members of the *B. melaninogenicus-oralis* group were much more sensitive to all three agents, for example *B. melaninogenicus* (15 strains) had MIC90s to cefotetan, cefoxitin and cefotaxime of 4, 2 and 1mg/litre respectively. All isolates were sensitive to metronidazole (range <0.12-2, MIC90=1mg/l) and clindamycin (range <0.12-8, MIC90=1 mg/l).

Cefotetan showed similar activity to cefoxitin and both were more active than cefotaxime. Cefotetan may prove useful in the treatment of *B. fragilis* infections where metronidazole is not appropriate.

References

1   Lode,H *et al* 1985. The role of pharmacokenitics in the clinical use of cephalosporins. In CEFOTETAN: a long acting antibiotic for poylmicrobial infections. H. Lode, P. Periti and C.J.L. Strachan (eds.). Churchill Livingstone, Edinburgh.

2   Murray, P.R. and Niles, A.C. 1983. Inoculum preparation for anaerobic susceptibility tests. J. Clin. Microbiol. 18: 733-734.

ABSTRACT   3

NCTC 11870: A NEW CONTROL ORGANISM FOR SUSCEPTIBILITY TESTING OF ANAEROBES

J.R. Edwards and P.J. Turner

ICI Pharmaceuticals Division, Mereside, Alderley Park, Macclesfield, Cheshire, SK10 4TG, England.

NCTC 11870 is a Beta-lactamase producing strain of *B.fragilis* which exhibits an excellent correlation between Minimum Inhibitory Concentration (MIC) values and disc susceptibility results. Using the well established Stokes method, this strain produces reliable results if an easily prepared standard inoculum is used. However, if the inoculum is too light, false sensitivity may be seen and conversely an excessively heavy inoculum may result in the zone being reduced in diameter or overgrown. This is demonstrated in the table 1 using cefotetan and cefotaxime:

Table.

Agent	MIC mg/l^{-1}	Correct	Inoculum Light	Heavy
		zone interpretation		
Cefotetan	16	S	S	R
Cefotaxime	64	R	S	R

The method is simple to perform and seems to be completely reliable for predicting susceptibility of anaerobes to Beta-lactam agents; wider use will establish its worth.

ABSTRACT 4

BIOCHEMICAL AND CHEMICAL STUDIES ON SOME POORLY CHARACTERISED, NON-FERMENTATIVE *BACTEROIDES* SPECIES

H.N. Shah and M.D. Collins*

Oral Microbiology, London Hospital Medical College, London, E1 2AD

* Department of Food Microbiology, Food Research Institute, Shinfield, Reading, RG2 9AT.

Bacteroides coagulans, *B. furcosus*, *B. pneumosintes*, *B. nodosus*, *B. praecutus*, *B. putredinus* and *B. ureolyticus* are non- or very weakly fermentative species whose DNA base composition (where known) range between 28 - 37 mol%

G+C. Although these organisms superficially appear to form a homogeneous group of 'atypical bacteroides', chemical and biochemical studies indicate they are taxonomically very diverse. Metabolic end-products, presumably in some cases derived from nitrogen metabolism, vary widely amongst these species. For example, *B. ureolyticus* produces major amounts of acetic and succinic acids, *B. putredinus* produces succinic, propionic and iso-valeric acids, whereas *B. preacutus* produces acetic, butyric and iso-valeric acids. The other species produce low levels of acetic acid and complex mixtures of other acids. Preliminary enzymatic studies also indicate considerable heterogeneity within this group. True bacteroides (the '*B. fragilis* group' of organisms) contain the pentose phosphate pathway enzymes, 6-phosphogluconate dehydrogenase (6PGDH) and glucose-6-phosphate dehydrogenase (G6PDH), together with malate and glutamate dehydrogenases (MDH and GDH respectively). None of the above species so far examined contain all of these enzymes. For example *B. coagulans* contains only GDH, *B. furcosus* an NADP dependent G6PDH while *B.preacutus* possess an NAD dependent 6PGDH.

The above non-fermentative 'bacteroides' species also exhibit considerable diversity in lipid composition. Thus the long chain fatty acids of *B. coagulans*, *B. furcosus* and *B. ureolyticus* are primarily of the straight-chain saturated and monounsaturated types, with hexadecanoic acid ($C_{16:0}$), octadecanoic acid ($C_{18:0}$) and octadecenoic (C_{18-1}) acids predominating. In contrast, the long chain fatty acids of *B. praecutus* and *B. putridinus* are primarily of the methyl-branched chain types, with 13-methyltetradecanoic (*iso*-C_{15-0}) acid predominating. These fatty acid patterns are quite distinct from those of true bacteroides (i.e. 'B. fragilis group') which also possess major amounts of methyl-branched chain acids but with 12-methyltetradecanoic (anteiso-$C_{15:0}$) acid predominating.

The present studies highlight the marked differences between these non-fermentative species and the 'B. fragilis group' of organisms and further emphasise the need to exclude these taxa from the genus Bacteroides.

ABSTRACT 5

INHIBITION BY BACTEROIDES VULGATUS AND ZYMOSAN OF THE KILLING OF ESCHERICHIA COLI BY POLYMORPHONUCLEAR LEUKOCYTES.

W.A.C. Vel, F. Namavar, A.M.J.J. Verweij, A.N.B. Pubben and D.M. MacLaren.

Research Group for Commensal Infections, Department of Medical Microbiology, School of Medicine, Vrije Universiteit, P.O.Box 7161, 1007 MC Amsterdam, The Netherlands.

The inhibition of phagocytosis and killing in vitro of facultative bacteria by polymorphonuclear leukocytes (PMNL) has been described as a property peculiar to anaerobes, mediated by their greater or more rapid binding of serum opsonins, in particular complement, and provides a possible explanation for the synergy observed in mixed aerobic/anaerobic infections. Literature on this subject recently has been reviewed by MacLaren et al.(2). To determine whether other complement depleting organisms are equally capable of inhibiting the killing of Escherichia coli, and whether competition for complement is the only mechanism involved, we compared the influence of

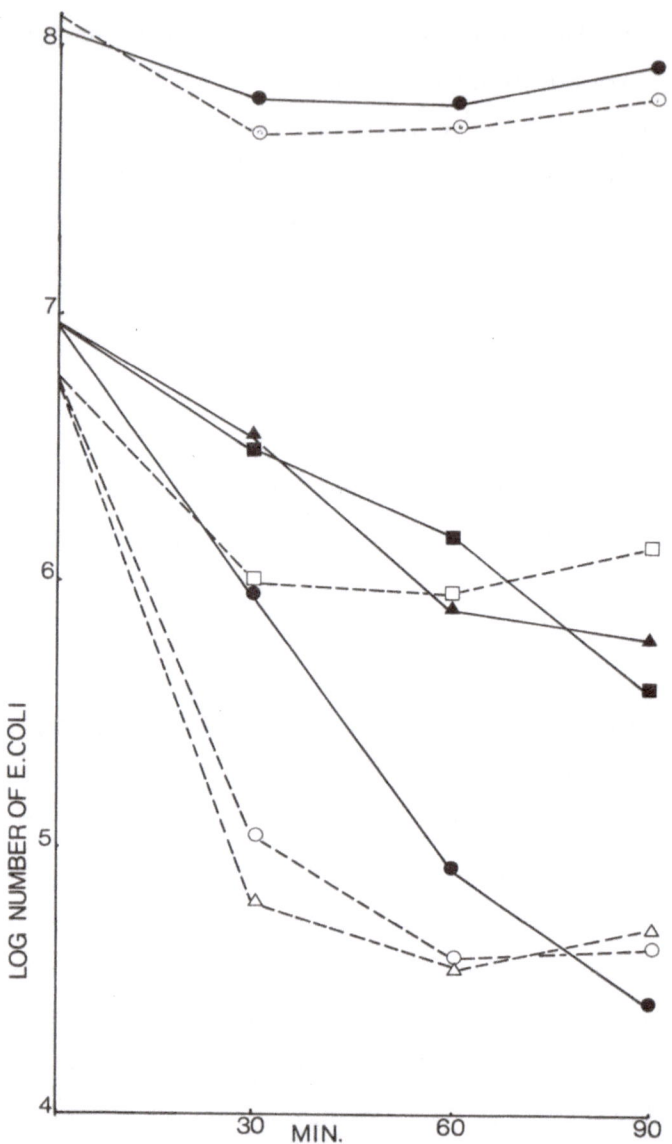

Figure 1. Effect of the presence of *B. vulgatus* or Zymosan and of the size of the inoculum on the killing of *E. coli* by PMNL. Solid lines: killing of *E. coli* by 5×10^6 PMNL/ml in the presence of 10% pooled normal human serum. ● : *E. coli* alone , ▲ : in the presence of 10^7 *B. vulgatus*/ml, ■ : in the presence of 10^7 Zymosan/ml. Dashed lines: killing of preopsonised *E. coli* by 5×10^6 PMNL/ml: ○ : alone, △ : in the presence of 10^7 preopsonised *B. vulgatus*/ml, □ : in the presence of 10^7 preopsonised Zymosan/ml. Values represent the mean log number of viable *E.coli* after lysis of the PMNL of at least three experiments.

Bacteroides vulgatus and of Zymosan on the killing of *E.coli* by human PMNL. *B. vulgatus* consumed complement rapidly, but was hardly killed itself: after 30 min. incubation it depleted serum of 98% of the complement haemolytic activity but only 20% of the inoculum was killed by that time (methods described by Vel et al.(3)). From many studies it is known that Zymosan is rapidly opsonised and phagocytosed. Neither *B.vulgatus* nor *E.coli* were sensitive to 10% pooled normal human serum. The figure shows that in the presence of 10% serum both *B.vulgatus* and Zymosan inhibited the killing of *E. coli* significantly (p<0.01, Wilcoxon signed rank test). When competition for complement was ruled out as a possible mechanism by pre-opsonisation of *E. coli*, *B. vulgatus* and Zymosan, only the latter had a significant inhibitory effect on the killing of *E. coli* (p<0.01). The figure also shows that when the inoculum of *E. coli* was increased, a larger proportion resisted killing. These results show that inhibition of the killing *in vitro* can result from a competition for complement which is not peculiar to anaerobes, and from saturation of the PMNL by organisms or particles which are phagocytosed themselves. They confirm similar observations by other authors (1). However nonspecific the inhibition of *in vitro* killing may be, the fact that some anaerobes compete for complement without being eliminated subsequently may be an important factor in the pathogenesis of mixed infections with these bacteria.

References

1   Dijkmans, B.A.C., Leijh, P.C.J, Braat, A.G.P. and van
     Furth, R. 1985. Effect of bacterial competition in
     the opsonisation, phagocytosis and intracellular
     killing of microorganisms by granulocytes.
     Infect. Immun. 49: 219-224.

2   MacLaren, D.M., Namavar, F., Verweij-van Vught,
     A.M.J.J, Vel, W.A.C. and Kaan, J.A. 1984.
     Pathogenic synergy: mixed intra-abdominal infections.
     Antonie van Leeuwenhoek 50: 775-787.

3   Vel, W.A.C., Namavar, F., Verweij-van Vught,
     A.M.J.J., Pubben, A.N.B. and MacLaren, D.M. 1985.
     Killing of *Escherichia coli* by human
     polymorphonuclear leukocytes in the presence of
     Bacteroides fragilis. J. Clin. Pathol. 38: 86-91.

ABSTRACT   6

THE USE OF FAST PROTEIN LIQUID CHROMATOGRAPHY FOR THE

IDENTIFICATION OF ANAEROBIC BACTERIA

S.P. Borriello, P.J. Reed and Fiona E. Barclay,

Division of Communicable Diseases, Clinical Research
Centre, Watford Road, Harrow, Middlesex, HA1 3UJ, UK.

The analysis of microbial cellular proteins by SDS-
polyacrylamide gel electrophoresis (PAGE) is increasingly

being used as a method of identifying and biotyping

bacteria.   The major limitation of SDS-PAGE is the diffi-

culty of interpreting and comparing the protein bands

generated.   Although coupling SDS-PAGE to laser densi-

tometry can help overcome this problem, it is not a

facility readily available.   We have devised a simple

procedure based on Fast Protein Liquid Chromatography

(FPLC) for generating protein profiles from bacteria.

Using this procedure we have grouped bacteria into

genera, species and, in some cases, sub-species by

profiling their native proteins.   The FPLC technique,

which is based on ion-exchange chromatography, analyses

simply prepared protein samples in about 20 minutes using

a salt gradient to elute bound material.   The resulting

trace is similar in many ways to the volatile fatty acid

profiles produced by gas-liquid chromatographic analysis of anaerobic cultures. In this case the peaks representing protein can be specified by the percentage salt concentration at which they elute.

Organisms to be identified are grown overnight in brain heart infusion broth, centrifuged at 4000 rpm for 20 min, the pellet washed in an equal volume of isotonic saline and the resultant pellet resuspended in de-ionised water to one tenth of the original volume. The cells are disrupted by freeze-thawing three times (liquid nitrogen or -30°C. to room temperature) and the cellular debris removed by centrifugation and filtration (0.2 micron). The protein content of the filtrate is estimated by the "Bio-Rad" protein assay, the sample adjusted to approx 1 mg of protein/ml by addition of deionised water and 200 microlitres injected onto the FPLC column.

The potential of the technique for identifying anaerobes is illustrated in the figure. We have recently

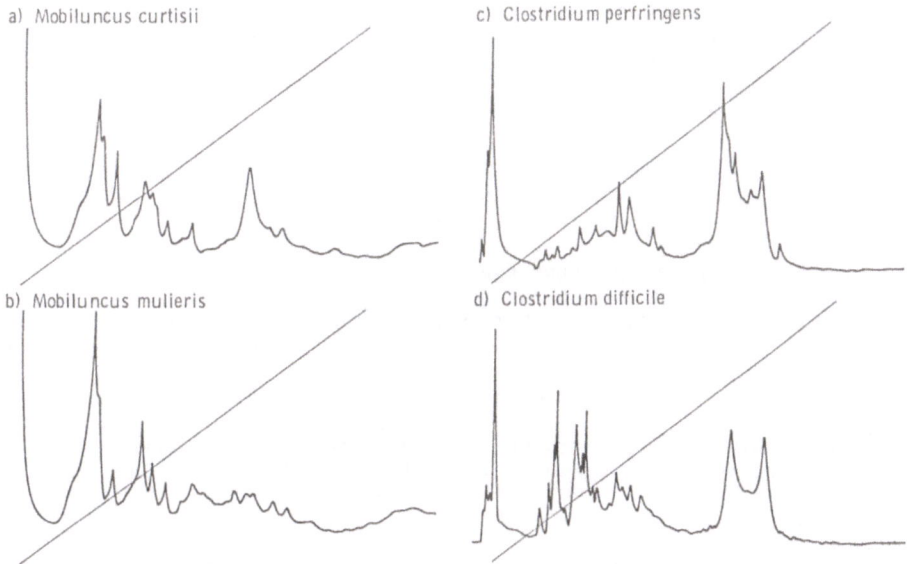

a) Mobiluncus curtisii

b) Mobiluncus mulieris

c) Clostridium perfringens

d) Clostridium difficile

shown that the FPLC profiles of *Bacteroides pentosaceus,*
B. capillus and *B. buccae* were indistinguishable, which
is of interest as these three species have been shown to
be synonymous (2).

By virtue of the simplicity of preparation of samples
and the robustness of the analytical columns this
technique overcomes many of the problems associated with
PAGE analysis. Profiles are reproducible on repeated
analysis of single samples and on duplicate preparation of
strains and characteristic profiles are not restricted to
anaerobic organisms (1). The results imply that FPLC may
be used to quickly and simply produce protein profiles to
identify bacteria to species or sub-species levels from a
single analysis.

References

1   Borriello, S. P., Reed, P. J. and Barclay, F. E.
     1985. Identification of bacteria by fast protein
     liquid chromatography. J. Med. Microbiol, 19: ix.

2   Johnson, J. L. and Holdeman, L. V. 1985.
     Bacteroides capillus Kornman and Holt and *Bacteroides*
     pentosaceus Shah and Collins, Later synonyms of
     Bacteroides buccae Holdeman *et al.*
     Int. J. Syst. Bacteriol. 35: 114.

ABSTRACT 7

MICROTUBE PLATE PROCEDURE FOR BIOCHEMICAL CHARACTERIZATION AND
ANTIMICROBIAL SUSCEPTIBILITY TESTING OF ANAEROBIC BACTERIA.

S.D. Allen, J.A. Siders, N.B. O'Bryan and E.H. Gerlach

Indiana University School of Medicine, Indianapolis,
IN 46223, and St. Francis Hospital, Wichita, KS 67214,
USA.

In 1982, we reported our initial development of a new
system for testing of anaerobic bacteria in microdilution

trays (1). The purpose of this report was to present an update of the system with a description of its current performance. The microtube plates are prepared by dispensing differential test substrates into 96-well microtiter plates by use of an automated Quick Spense dispensing device (Bellco Laboratories, Inc.). Each bio-chemical plate includes 43 differential tests. In addition, varying concentrations of antimicrobial agents are prepared in Wilkins-Chalgren broth (Difco Laboratories) and dispensed into the plates. The plates are stored at $-80°C$.; prior to use, they are thawed and held in an anaerobic chamber for 4 h. For inoculation, pure cultures are grown overnight in Schaedler broth (BBL). Following incubation, turbid broth cultures are diluted to a McFarland No. 1 turbidity standard and further diluted 1:10 in sterile water (containing 0.02% tween 80). The trays are inoculated (in air) using plastic replicators then incubated anaerobically for 24-48 h. New software programs were developed for archival, retrieval and numerical identification using a large main-frame DEC-20 computer. The computer-stored data base includes Gram-reaction, morphology, volatile acid-metabolic products (determined using gas-liquid chromatography GLC), fermentation reactions, growth in presence of certain antibiotics and other differential tests. More than 6000 bacteria are now in the data base; they include ATCC, CDC and other reference strains, fresh clinical isolates and fecal flora isolates that were all characterized simulta-neously using conventional reference laboratory procedures. In the evaluation phase of the study, consecutively encountered fresh clinical isolates were identified using the microtiter system and accuracy of identifications was determined by comparing results with identifications obtained using conventional VPI procedures (2).

Without additional tests, the identification accuracy of the system, which consisted of the microtiter plate differential tests, plus Gram-stain features and GLC results, correctly identified 87% of 549 fresh clinical isolates. With a few additional supplemental tests, such as reactions on egg yolk agar, gelatin hydrolysis, and action on milk, accuracy improved to an overall 97% (532/549) for specific identification.

We have found the system to be useful for both research and clinical diagnostic applications. With the computer terminal in our laboratory, the numerical profile number that we assign to each isolate, based on differential test results, permits rapid interpretation of data and identification of individual isolates. The major advantage of this system is its relatively low materials cost and personnel time savings because of the automation and rapid data processing capability. In our laboratory, two microbiologists can test approximately 200 anaerobe isolates per day on a large battery of differential test substrates and against multiple antimicrobics in varying dilution series.

References

1   Allen, S.D., J.A. Siders, Johnson, K.S. and E.H. Gerlach. 1982. Biochemical characterization and antimicrobial susceptibility testing of anaerobic bacteria in microdilution trays. In: R.C. Tilton (ed.), Rapid methods and automation in microbiology. American Society for Microbiology, Washington, D.C. p. 266-270.

2   Holdeman, L.V., Cato, E.P. and Moore, W.E.C. (eds.). 1977. Anaerobe laboratory manual, 4th ed. Virginia Polytechnic Institute and State University, Blacksburg, VA.

ABSTRACT 8

FAECAL ANAEROBE FLORA AND FEACAL VITAMIN K CONCENTRATIONS IN RESPONSE TO DIET AND ANTIMICROBIAL AGENTS: INVESTIGATIONS WITH MOXALACTAM, CEFOPERAZONE AND CLINDAMYCIN

S.D. Allen, J.A. Siders, C.G. Kindberg, P.M. Allison, N.U. Bang, M.D. Cromer, N.B. O'Bryan, G.L. Brier, and J.H. Suttie.

Indiana University School of Medicine, Indianapolis, IN; University of Wisconsin, Madison, WI; and Lilly Laboratory for Clinical Research, Indianapolis, IN, USA.

It has been postulated that vitamin K deficiency may result from inadequate dietary intake of vitamin K_1, also called phylloquinone (present in various plants consumed in the diet) and from decreased synthesis of bacterial menaquinones (vitamin K_2 compounds) caused by the action of broad-spectrum antibiotics in the gastrointestinal tract. Although it has been established that starvation alone does not induce hypoprothrombinemia and a bleeding tendency in patients unless antibiotics are received concomitantly, the role of the intestinal microbiota in production of menaquinones within the gut and their importance in coagulation homeostasis has not been demonstrated.

The purpose of this report was to present data on the effects of moxalactam (MOX), cefoperazone (CPZ) and clindamycin (CLM) on the faecal flora and faecal menaquinone and phylloquinone concentrations of volunteers who received a vitamin K-deficient diet. MOX and CPZ are 3rd generation beta-lactam compounds which differ in their structures, spectra of activity and modes of action from CLM. All 3 agents are excreted in bile in high concentration and are active against many anaerobes.

The volunteers were healthy males, ages 21 to 50; each received a partially defined diet (Sustacal, Mead Johnson & Co.), mixed with skimmed-milk, that was nutritionally complete, except that the diet lacked vitamin K. Three groups of 3 volunteers received MOX 4g, CPZ 8g and CLM 2.4g i.v. in divided doses each day for ten days. On days 0, 2-3 and 10, the feacal anaerobic and aerobic flora was determined quantitatively using selective and nonselective media and isolation procedures. Anaerobic processing of specimens and incubation was done in an anaerobic chamber. Isolates were definitively identified to species using conventional reference methods. Chloroform/methanol extracts of the stool specimens were analyzed for K and MK compounds using reverse-phase HPLC.

Decreased MK levels were found with MOX (1/3), CPZ (3/3) and CLM 3/3 volunteers) and showed a direct correlation with reduced numbers of certain anaerobe species, particularly of the *Bacteroides fragilis* group and certain Gram-positive anaerobes. The predominant faecal menaquinone was MK-10. Species of *Bacteroides* are probably the numerically dominant producers of MK-10 within the gut. MK-8, which is produced by facultative anaerobes including *Escherichia coli* and certain streptococci, was not a major menaquinone within faeces of these healthy humans.

The marked decrease in faecal menaquinone levels in the cefoperazone and clindamycin groups may be attributed to the profound antimicrobial activities of these compounds against the anaerobic flora. There was a varied response in the faecal anaerobic flora and MK levels of subjects who received moxalactam. Previously, we found that moxalactam in a higher dose (6g/day) eliminated the *B. fragilis* group from 4 of 5 subjects (1). This dose-dependent effect of moxalactam on the anaerobic flora may have potential clinical significance.

Although menaquinone synthesis by the intestinal flora, particularly the anaerobic component, may play a role in vitamin K-dependent clotting homeostasis of individuals whose diets lack vitamin K, further work is needed to determine whether menaquinones are absorbed through the intestinal tract and their bioactivity within extra-intestinal tissue of humans.

Reference

1 Allen, S.D., Siders, J.A., Cromer,M.D., Fischer,J.A., Smith, J.W. and Israel K.S. 1980. Effect of LY127935 (6059-S) on human fecal flora. Proceedings of the 11th international congress of chemotherapy, American Society for Microbiology, Washington, D.C. p. 101-103.

ABSTRACT 9

COMPOSITION OF BACTERIAL FLORA IN ILEAL RESERVOIR PATIENTS

M.D. Holdom, M.J. Hill, R.L. Moskowitz and R.J. Nicholls

PHLS-CAMR, SALISBURY, Wiltshire, UK. and
St Marks Hospital, City Road, LONDON, UK.

A proctocolectomy with ileal reservoir and anal anastomosis was described by Parks and Nicholls (3). The colon and upper half of the rectum are removed along with any other inflamed rectal stump mucosa. A reservoir is constructed from the terminal ileum drawn down through the divided rectum and an anastomosis performed.

While most patients have satisfactory functional results, reservoir inflammation has been observed in some patients. The aim of this study was to analyse the bacterial flora from the reservoir and to relate it to the presence or absence of inflammation in these patients, with a view to finding any possible bacteriological cause for the symptoms. Comparison was made of the reservoir floras of patients who originally had ulcerative colitis with those who had polyposis. Varying reservoir constructions (S-reservoir J-reservoir, and W-reservoir) were studied to highlight any differences between them.

Bacterial count determinations were performed using a semi-quantitive streaking method which was calibrated by initial Miles, Misra and Irwin quantitive methods (1). The method used seventeen selective and non-selective media. Bacterial genera were identified using sub-culture and microscopic techniques.

Results show that the reservoir flora has bacterial counts which fall between that of ileostomies and normal faecal flora.

Significantly higher levels in the inflammation patients, compared to the healthy reservoir patients, of total aerobes and yeasts are seen. The rise in aerobic bacteria in these patients agree with the findings of Nicholls *et al* (2). Large rises in the *Bifidobacterium* sp, *Clostridium* sp. and *Veillonella* sp. counts were also seen.

No significant differences were seen between the floras of polyposis and ulcerative colitics who underwent the same operation. Anaerobic counts appear to be lowered in the polyposis patients compared to the ulcerative colitis group, although *Bacteroides* sp. and *Lactobacillus* sp. were increased in polyposis.

Results suggest that the S-reservoir construction may harbour higher numbers of anaerobic bacteria, with signif-icantly higher counts of *Bacteroides fragilis* group, while the J-reservoir appears to have the higher numbers of aerobes.

The fact that the pathogens looked for were not seen (although *Shigella* and *Salmonella* sp. were not actively looked for) suggests that a change in the bacterial profile either due to some change in the environment allowing changes in dominant organisms or metabolic changes within bacteria which could produce causative inflammatory agents

References

1   Miles, A.A., Misra, S.S. and Irwin, J.O. 1938. The estimation of the bactericidal power of the blood. J. Hyg. 38: 732-749.

2   Nicholls, R.J., Belliveau, P., Neill, M., Wilks, M. and Tabaqchali, S. 1981. Restorative proctocolectomy with ileal reservoir: a paraphysiological assessment. Gut 22: 462-468.

3   Parks, A.G. and Nicholls, R.J. 1978. Proctocolectomy without ileostomy for ulcerative colitis. Brit. Med. Journal 2: 85-88.

ABSTRACT 10

FOOD INTOLERANCE AND MICROBIAL POPULATIONS IN THE HUMAN COLON

Hazel K.Bradley[1], Catherine E. Bayliss[1], G.M. Wyatt[1], Anne F. Smith[1], Virginia A. Jones and J.O. Hunter.

[1] AFRC Food Research Institute, Colney Lane, Norwich NR4 7UA, U.K. Department of Gastroenterology, Addenbrookes Hospital, Cambridge, U.K.

Food intolerance is a major factor in Irritable Bowel Syndrome. The association between food and symptoms has been tested in a number of patients (1). Several observations point to the significance of the bacterial flora in this phenomenon:

* 11/88 patients dated symptoms from a gut infection

* A further 10/88 patients dated symptoms from a course of antibiotics

* 13/88 dated symptoms from abdominal or pelvic surgery
* In a prospective trial with 128 patients undergoing hysterectomy 16.2% of those receiving prophylactic metronidazole were suffering symptoms of IBS six weeks post operatively, while only 2.5% of those not receiving metronidazole complained of symptoms (2)
* Food challenge in these patients did not produce the symptoms of pain, flatulence and sometimes diarrhoea until 16-72h after challenge.

   In preliminary experiments six patients were hospitalised and analysis of the faecal flora was carried out for 48h before and 72h after challenge with wheat (5 patients) or sugar (1 patient) (3).

Results suggested:

* Higher numbers of facultative organisms in patients than in controls
* Mucoid and palisade - forming Gram-negative aerobes isolated in higher numbers in patients

Subsequently, three detailed studies were carried out:

a) In a large scale blind study, a total of 103 stool samples from 101 patients and controls have been examined for levels and types of facultative bacteria. A subgroup of 35 female samples were patients and controls from a hysterectomy study. Some subjects had received metronidazole prophylactically, but others had received treatment courses with a range of antibiotics. The levels of facultative bacteria recovered from antibiotic treated patients and controls were higher than from groups receiving prophylactic metronidazole or no antibiotic treatment. The difference was significant for the control groups ($p < 0.05$). All other groupings of patients and controls did not show significant differences. The proportion of Gram-positive organisms present in the IBS group was lower than in the control group but the differences were not significant, but increased recovery of *Enterobacteriaceae* was a feature of all the antibiotic and non-antibiotic patient groups although none of the differences were significant.

b) Four patients were challenged on several consecutive days during a 10 day hospitalisation period and obligate and facultative faecal floras analysed. Incorrect diagnosis and unconnected symptoms led to the rejection of data from two patients. The levels of anaerobes were generally stable before, during and after challenge; however the species were unstable. Instability in the facultative populations was noted during the period of challenge, in particular in the numbers of lactobacilli.

c) The flora of one patient with multiple intolerances and showing severe symptoms, and whose extensive drug treatment included 9 antibiotics, was analysed at intervals over a two year period. Her flora was exceptionally unstable, being at times almost wholly facultative and at other times completely dominated by *Clostridium* spp. No marked correlation was seen between the pattern of antibiotic resistance of isolates, administration of the drugs or severity of symptoms.

Clearly there are alterations in the microbial flora of the large bowel in some of the IBS patients studied.

Hazel Bradley and Anne Smyth were supported by a grant from the East Anglian Regional Health Authority.

References

1   A. Jones, V., McLaughlan, P., Shirthouse, M., Workman, E. and Hunter, J.O. 1982. Lancet 8308: 1115-1117.

304

2   A. Jones, V., Wilson, A.J., Hunter, J.O. and
     Robinson, R.E. 1984. J. Obstet. Gynaecol. 5 (Suppl.
     1): S22-23.

3   Bayliss, C.E., Houston, A.P., A. Jones, V., Hishon,
     S. and Hunter, J.O. 1984. Proc. Nut. Soc. 43: 16A.

ABSTRACT   11

IMPACT   OF DIFFERENT ANTIMICROBIAL AGENTS ON THE ANAEROBIC

OROPHARYNGEAL AND INTESTINAL MICROFLORA

C.E. Nord and A. Heimdahl

Departments of Microbiology and Oral Surgery, Huddinge
University Hospital, Karolinska Institute and National
Bacteriological Laboratory, Stockholm, Sweden.

The   normal   human gastrointestinal   microflora   is   a
stable   ecosystem.   When physiological or ecological
disturbances take place in the digestive tract, changes in
the microflora can be found.   The most common cause of
disturbances in the normal human microflora is the administration of antimicrobials (1). In this abstract we report
our experience from investigations of the impact of
different antimicrobial agents on the anaerobic oropharyngeal and intestinal microflora.

    Phenoxymethylpenicillin,   bacampicillin,   cefaclor,
clindamycin,   erythromycin and doxycycline were given
perorally to a total of 52 subjects during seven days. The
numbers of aerobic and anaerobic bacteria in the oropharyngeal
and intestinal microflora were determined, as were the
concentrations of antimicrobial agents in the oropharyngeal
and intestinal tracts. Clindamycin, erythromycin and doxycycline
were detected in both saliva and faeces. Phenoxy-methylpenicillin,
bacampicillin, cefaclor and doxycycline caused only minor

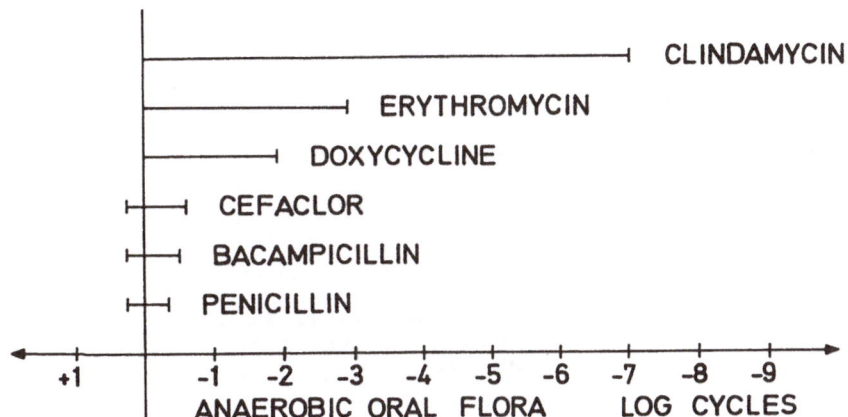

Figure 1. Changes caused by different antimicrobial agents in total colony counts ($\log_{10}$) of the anaerobic oropharyngeal microflora. The horizontal lines indicate the changes expressed as mean values of the total colony count obtained.
+ = increase in numbers of microorganisms.
− = decrease in numbers of microorganisms.

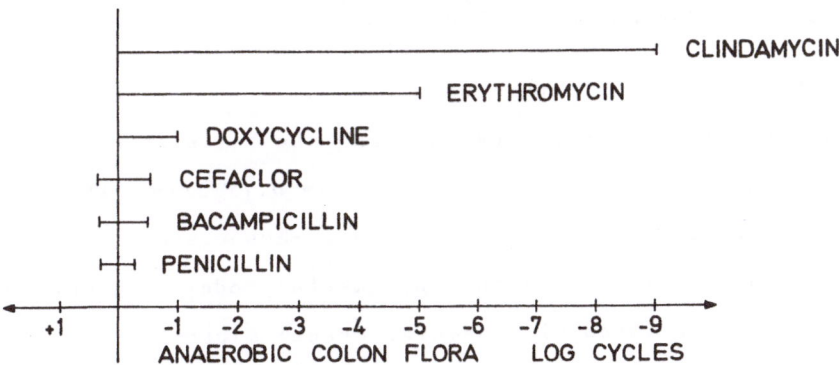

Figure 2. Changes caused by different antimicrobial agents in total colony counts ($\log_{10}$) of the anaerobic colon microflora.

changes in the microflora, while pronounced suppression of anaerobic bacteria was noticed when clindamycin was administered. (Figures 1 and 2). Erythromycin decreased the aerobic bacteria in the oropharynx and both aerobic and anaerobic bacteria in the colon. New colonizing clostridia, enterobacteria and fungi were found in both the oropharynx and colon when erythromycin and clindamycin were administered.

Reference

1   Nord, C.E., Kager,L. and Heimdahl, A. 1984. The impact of anti-microbials and the risk of infections. Amer. J. Med. 76: 99-106.

ABSTRACT   12

COLONIZATION RESISTANCE TO *CLOSTRIDIUM DIFFICILE* : EVALUATION OF VOLATILE FATTY ACID CONCENTRATION IN CAECAL CONTENTS FROM DIFFERENT TYPES OF ANIMALS

W.J. Su*, M.J. Waechter, M. Dolegeal, P. Bourlioux* and G. Mahuzier

Laboratoires de Microbiologie* et Chimie Analytique, Faculte de Pharmacie, 92 290 - Chatenay-Malabry, FRANCE

The purpose of this work was to study the role of volatile fatty acids (VFAs) in the resistance to intestinal colonization by *Clostridium difficile*, that is the agent implicated in antibiotic-associated pseudo-membranous colitis, in an experimental model of germfree (GF) mice associated with hamster caecal micro-flora.

First, the colonization resistance to *C. difficile* was verified in conventional hamsters. Then hamster caecal

Table. Colonization resistance to *Clostridium difficile* and concentrations of Volatile Fatty Acids in ceacal contents.

	Number of animals	Colonization resistance	*C. difficile* per g of faeces	eq of Volatile Fatty acid per g of ceacal contents (wet weight)					
				acetic	propionic	isobutyric	butyric	isovaleric	valeric
Coventional Hamsters	6	+	<10^2	94.8* ± 19.6	13.2 ± 3.29	0.42 ± 0.11	15.9 ± 5.06	0.25 ± 0.08	1.66 ± 0.69
Germfree Mice	7	–	–	5.54 ± 2.86	ND**	ND	ND	ND	ND
GF Mice with *C. difficile*	7	–	10^8–10^9	12.1 ± 2.03	0.11 ± 0.02	0.17 ± 0.10	0.24 ± 0.21	0.13 ± 0.05	Trace
Mice Group 1	9	+	<10^2	45.5 ± 14.0	5.68 ± 2.41	0.19 ± 0.08	16.0 ± 9.56	0.19 ± 0.09	0.09 ± 0.03
Mice Group 2	9	+	<10^2	46.9 ± 5.84	1.12 ± 0.45	0.2 ± 0.11	20.0 ± 10.1	0.22 ± 0.16	0.10 ± 0.01
Mice Group 3	6	partial	10^6–10^7	42.5 ± 14.0	5.23 ± 2.56	0.22 ± 0.16	10.2 ± 4.42	0.17 ± 0.12	0.1 ± 0.01

* mean + SD
** Not detectable

flora was transferred to C₃H GF mice orally. After treatment with erythromycin, the colonization resistance is always maintained (group 1). Heating (70°C/10 min) of 10^{-2} dilution of caecal contents from mice of group 1 was performed to simplify the microflora as well as to maintain colonization resistance (group 2). Another group of GF mice was inoculated with an anaerobic culture of 10^{-6} dilution of heated caecal microflora, the population of C.difficile was maintained $10^6 - 10^7$ CFU/g of faeces (group 3).

The VFA concentrations were evaluated in caecal contents from GF mice, GF mice associated with C.difficile, GF mice associated with different microflora (groups 1, 2 and 3) and conventional hamsters by gas chromatography.

Only acetic acid (AA) was detected in the caecal contents of GF mice (AA), propionic acid (PA), isobutyric acid, butyric acid (BA), isovaleric acid and valeric acid were detected in the cecal contents of all other animal groups where the concentrations of AA, PA and BA were more important than the others. Furthermore, PA and BA were present in markedly increased quantities in the caecal contents of mice possessing colonization resistance or partial colonization resistance.

However, the MICs of AA, PA and BA *in vitro* against C.difficile were more than 200 mcg/ml (pH 6.8). The results suggest that the VFAs may play a role in colonization resistance to C. difficile but this resistance was not due to VFAs alone. Other mechanisms are likely to contribute.

ABSTRACT   13

IDENTIFICATION OF *CLOSTRIDIUM DIFFICILE* USING THE API ZYM SYSTEM.

P.N.Levett

PHLS Anaerobe Reference Unit, Luton LU4 0DZ, UK.

Efficient selective media are available for the isolation of *Clostridium difficile* from faecal specimens. However, these media are not absolutely selective for *C.difficile* and several clostridial species may be recovered (2), including *C.beijerinckii*, *C.paraputrificum* *C. butyricum*, *C. fallax*, *C. glycolicum*, *C. innocuum* and *C.bifermentans*, *C.perfringens*, *C.sporogenes* and *C.sordellii* may also be isolated on these media, but can readily be differentiated from *C. difficile* by their production of lecithinase or lipase.

Gas-liquid chromatography (GLC) may be used to identify *C. difficile* directly from the primary isolation medium (1,3). If GLC is not available, identification of suspected *C. difficile* by conventional methods is necessary and this may delay a final report by as much as five days.

The use of the API ZYM system for the identification of *C. difficile* and related clostridia was investigated. API ZYM strips contain enzyme-specific substrates, facilitating the semi-quantitative detection of 19 enzymes. This system further offers the potential advantages of aerobic incubation and a 4 hour incubation period. Using this system *C. difficile* was readily differentiated from other egg yolk-negative clostridia.

All strains of *C. difficile* produced strong activity of C4 esterase, C8 esterase and leucine arylamidase. *C.glycolicum* resembled *C. difficile* most closely, but was distinguished from *C. difficile* by strong activity of both acid and alkaline phosphatases.

The enzyme activity of *C. difficile* was found to vary depending upon the composition of the medium upon which the inoculum was grown. However, on a given medium the activity appeared to be constant. Brain heart infusion agar and Columbia agar were considered suitable basal media, to which was added 7% horse blood. A reduction of the incubation time to 24 hours provided a more rapid identification of *C. difficile*. In order to achieve a sufficiently heavy inoculum it was then necessary to harvest the growth from two or three plates.

The results of this study suggest that, given standardised conditions and adequate controls, the API ZYM system may be a suitably rapid alternative to conventional identification techniques for *C. difficile*, in those laboratories lacking the facilities for GLC.

References

1   Levett, P.N. and Phillips, K.D. 1985. Gas-
     chromatographic identification of *Clostridium
     difficile* and detection of cytotoxin from a modified
     selective medium. J. Clin. Pathol. 38: 82-85.

2   Phillips, K.D., Brazier, J.S., Levett, P.N. and
     Willis, A.T. 1985. Isolation and identification of
     clostridia. In: Collins, C.H. & Grange, J.M. (eds.),
     Society for Applied Bacteriology Technical Series
     vol. 21, London: Academic Press. pp.215-236.

3   Phillips, K.D. and Rogers, P.A. 1981. Rapid
     detection and presumptive identification of
     Clostridium difficile by p-cresol production on a
     selective medium. J. Clin. Pathol. 34: 642-644.

ABSTRACT 14

AN IMMUNOCHEMICAL FINGERPRINTING METHOD FOR *CLOSTRIDIUM DIFFICILE*

Jacqueline Sharp and I.R. Poxton.

Department of Bacteriology, University of Edinburgh
Medical School, Teviot Place, Edinburgh, EH8 9AG. UK.

The use of SDS-polyacrylamide gel electrophoresis
(SDS-PAGE) in association with electrophoretic transfer of
separated proteins to nitrocellulose and subsequent
probing with antiserum (raised to whole cells of
Clostridium difficile NCTC 11223) could be useful for
finger-printing *C. difficile* (1, Cumming *et al.*, unpublished
results). For successful use in epidemiological studies
of the organism, it was important to establish whether or
not the surface antigens being probed were stable both
during subculture and after EDTA treatment of cells.

Results have shown that the antigenic profile of any
individual strain remains remarkably stable both during
subculture on the bench and *in vivo* in a mouse model. It
has been demonstrated that minor differences in the
temperature used during the EDTA treatment and the
duration of antigen extraction do not markedly alter the
SDS-PAGE and immunoblot profiles produced. Freeze-thawing
of the preparations during antigen extraction resulted in
a more detailed SDS-PAGE pattern but no change in the
immunoblot pattern.

It has also been demonstrated that an individual may
harbour more than one strain of the organism at any one
time. This observation will further complicate studies on
the epidemiology of *C. difficile*-associated disease. It
is suggested that for any detailed investigation several
C. difficile colonies should be sub-cultured from the
primary isolation plate.

Reference

1   Poxton,I.R., Aronsson,B., Mollby,R., Ward,C.E. and
     Collee,J.G. 1984. Immunochemical fingerprinting of
     Clostridium difficile strains isolated from an
     outbreak of antibiotic-associated colitis and
     diarrhoea. J. Med. Microbiol. 17: 317-324.

ABSTRACT   15

IOTA TOXIN PRODUCED BY BOTH CLOSTRIDIUM SPIROFORME AND CLOSTRIDIUM

PERFRINGENS TYPE E IS A SYNERGISTIC COMBINATION OF TWO PROTEINS

R.J. Carman, B.G. Stiles and T.D. Wilkins

Department of Anaerobic Microbiology, Virginia Polytechnic
Institute and State University, Blacksburg, Va 24061,
U.S.A.

Clostridium spiroforme,   which causes an acute and   fatal

enterotoxaemia of rabbits at weaning and following   anti-

microbial therapy, and *C.perfringens* Type E, an infrequent

cause of scouring in livestock, both produce an   extra-

cellular toxin which can be neutralized by commercially

available antiserum to the iota toxin of *C. perfringens*.

They   each produce two common but unrelated protein

antigens which can be demonstrated in culture filtrates by

crossed   immunoelectrophoresis using our own antisera to

either species.   These two protein antigens were purified

to homogeneity and have been shown that together they make

up iota toxin.   We name them i$_a$ and i$_b$.   Our purification

scheme consisted of the following preparative techniques:

saturated ammonium sulphate precipitation,   DEAE   ion

exchange and phenyl sepharose hydrophobic   interaction

Table 1. Biological activity of purified ia and ib

Assay	C.spiroforme[1]	C.perfringens[2]
Mouse i.p.[3]		
ia (0.5 ml)	−	−
ib (0.5 ml)	−	−
ia + ib (0.25 ml each)	+	+
Guinea pig i.d.[4]		
ia (0.3 ml)	−	−
ib (0.3 ml)	−	−
ia + ib (0.15 ml each)	+	+
Rabbit ileal loop		
ia (1.0 ml)	−	Not done
ib (1.0 ml)	−	Not done
ia + ib (0.5 ml each)	+	Not done

1. ia − 2 ug/ml; ib − 18 ug/ml.
2. ia − 3 ug/ml; ib − 27 ug/ml.
3. i.p. = intraperitoneal
4. i.d. = intradermal

chromatography, isoelectric focusing, Sephadex G-100 gel filtration and flat bed electrophoresis. At each stage the recovery of ia and ib was monitered by fused rocket immunoelectrophoresis. The biological activities and physical characteristics of ia and ib are shown in Tables 1 and 2. Maximum biological activity occured only when

Table 2. Physical properties of purified iota toxin

Physical property	C.spiroforme		C.perfringens	
	ia	ib	ia	ib
Isoelectric point	5.3	4.6	5.2	4.2
Molecular weight*	45000	68000	48000	67000

* Measured by Sephadex G- 100 filtration

both molecules were mixed. However, either by themselves had slight activity, ib more than ia. Mixtures of both were lethal, dermonecrotic, cytotoxic and enterotoxic.

All these activities were neutralizable by antisera to either ia or ib.

ABSTRACT 16

THE USE OF BACTEROIDES FRAGILIS GROUP AS INDICATORS OF SEWAGE POLLUTION OF ENVIRONMENTAL WATERS

R.J. Carman,

Department of Applied Biology, University of Wales Institute of Science and Technology, King Edward VII Avenue, Cardiff CF1 3NU, Wales

The usefulness of the *Bacteroides fragilis* group (BFG), which consists of *B. distasonis*, *B. fragilis*, *B. ovatus*, *B. thetaiotaomicron* and *B. vulgatus*, as an indicator of sewage pollution of environmental water was assessed in comparison to the frequently used indicator, faecal coliforms (FC). Indicator strains were isolated using membrane filtration followed by culture on selective media (gentamicin and penicillin supplemented blood agar for BFG and 0.4% enriched Teepol broth for FC). BFG were incubated at $30°C$ for 4h followed by 36h at $37°C$, whilst FC was incubated at $30°C$ for 4h and then for 14h at $44°C$. The ratios of the BFG to FC in fresh human and pig faeces, sewage treatment works influent and effluent, river water upstream and downstream from a sewage plant and lastly in seawater nearby and removed from sewage outfall on the foreshore of a popular seaside resort were calculated (Table). The ratio in both types of faeces was over 45; in the environmental samples it ranged from 30 to 45. The BFG survived as well, if not better, than FC in filtered river water and seawater stored in the dark at $4°C$. If

Table.   Recovery of BFG and FC from various sources

Source	BFG*	FC*	FG:FC
Human faeces	2.0×10^8	2.1×10^6	95
Pig faeces	2.3×10^8	5.1×10^6	45
Sewage influent**	2.8×10^8	6.1×10^6	46
Sewage effluent	4.4×10^6	1.5×10^5	30
River (700m upstream from plant)	2.7×10^3	8.9×10^1	30
River (4.8km downstream from plant)	3.2×10^5	9.0×10^3	36
Seawater (20m from outfall)	1.4×10^5	4.6×10^3	30
Seawater (800m from outfall)	1.6×10^5	5.2×10^3	31

*All counts are the mean of five and are expressed as counts/100ml.
**Domestic imput to percolating filter plant, little or no
industrial or agricultural waste.
BFG ARE UP TO 30 FOLD MORE FREQUENT IN ENVIRONMENTAL WATERS THAN FC

the isolation and identification methods for the BFG could
be made faster and cheaper, its relatively higher
frequency of isolation would make it a good indicator of
sewage pollution.

ABSTRACT   17

ANAEROBE HOLDING CHAMBER

J.D. Brown and Wendy J. Smith.

Microbiology Department, The General Hospital, Birmingham, UK.

The use of a holding chamber or jar utilising a flow
of nitrogen to maintain reduced oxygen levels was
described by Martin in 1971 (2).   Recently a prototype

anaerobe holding chamber of new design was produced by
(Don Whitley Ltd., Shipley, Yorkshire, UK.), consisting of
a Plexiglass box with a hinged lid, measuring 360 x 230 x
250 mm high, and having two gas flow rates, set at six
litres/min. and 400 ml/min., for the evaluation. When
flushed with nitrogen at the higher rate for five minutes,
followed by a constant flow at the lower rate, an oxygen
level of approximately 1% is obtained.

Viable counts of a range of anaerobic bacteria were
compared following immediate incubation and holding times
of up to seven hours in air and in the holding chamber.

Specimens from patients suspected of having an anaerobic infection were plated in triplicate on blood agar,
nalidixic acid Tween 80 blood agar (3), and kanamycin
menadione blood agar (1). One set was incubated immediately in the anaerobic cabinet, one set held in the
holding chamber, and the third set held in air until the
end of the working day.

Freshly isolated strains of *Clostridium perfringens*
and *Bacteroides fragilis* showed no significant differences
in the viable counts between the plates held in air and
those held in the holding chamber. Laboratory collection
strains of *C. novyi* type A and *C. butyricum*, and freshly
isolated strains of *Peptococcus* spp. and *B. oralis* showed
a reduction in viable counts on those plates held on the
bench compared with those held in the holding chamber.

The viable counts of *C. butyricum* and *Peptococcus* spp.
were unchanged after six hours. in the holding box, but
dropped by 50% after five hours storage in air. *C. novyi*
type A showed only a slight drop between four and seven
hours in the holding chamber. Those plates held in air
showed a drop of 50% after six hours. *B. oralis* held the

initial count for three hours in the holding chamber, and dropped by 25% after five hours. The plates held in air showed a drop of 50% after two hours, and produced no growth after five hours.

From 40 patients specimens examined, 12 yielded anaerobic organisms, and 11 of these gave exactly the same results on all 3 sets of plates. One specimen produced a very light growth of *Peptococcus* spp. on the plates incubated immediately and those held in air. This was not reported from those held in the holding chamber.

The viable count study indicated that the anaerobe holding chamber would be of no benefit in the isolation of the common anaerobes, *C. perfringens* and *B. fragilis*, but might prove to be useful in the isolation of less common anaerobes from clinical specimens. The clinical trial results are somewhat disappointing, but the number of specimens examined is too small to assess whether the holding chamber increases the isolation rate of less common anaerobes. The trial is still proceeding.

References

1   Dowell, V.R. and Hawkins, T.M. 1974 Laboratory
     methods in anaerobic bacteriology. C.D.C. Laboratory
     Manual P. 54.

2   Martin, W.J. 1971. Practical method for isolation
     of anaerobic bacteria in the clinical laboratory.
     Appl. Microbiol. 22: 1168-1171.

3   Wren, M.W.D. 1978. A new selective medium for the
     isolation of non-sporing anaerobic bacteria from
     clinical specimens.
     Medical Laboratory Sciences 35: 371-378.

ABSTRACT 18

ISOLATION OF ANAEROBES IN THE ROUTINE LABORATORY

K.W. Bennett and B.I. Duerden*

Departments of Bacteriology, Royal Hallamshire Hospital and *Medical Microbiology, University of Sheffield Medical School.

Laboratory diagnosis of anaerobic infections requires effective selective media for the isolation of anaerobes from mixed cultures, and a reliable system of anaerobic incubation. We performed quantitative and qualitative studies with a wide range of common pathogenic anaerobes on non-selective Columbia horse blood agar (CBA), both fresh and pre-reduced, and on three selective media containing nalidixic acid 10mg/L as the selective agent – CBA (NEG), and Wilkins- Chalgren agar with (NAT) and without (NAL) 0.1% Tween 80 – each incubated in an anaerobic jar and an anaerobic cabinet. For the quantitative study, broth cultures of reference strains and clinical isolates of fusobacteria (10 strains), pigmented bacteroides (3), *Bacteroides ureolyticus* (3), leptotrichia (1), clostridia (10) and anaerobic cocci (12) were serially diluted in a reduced diluent (RD) and 0.02ml plated onto the test media. In the qualitative study, clinical specimens on swabs were expressed in RD and a loopful plated on the media. Duplicate sets of media were incubated in an anaerobic jar and in a Whitley anaerobic cabinet, both with an atmosphere of $N_2:80\%$, $H_2:10\%$, $CO_2:10\%$.

There were no differences between the isolation rates (qualitative) or the quantitative recoveries of any of the anaerobes after incubation in jars with fresh or pre-reduced media or in the cabinet. With some isolates, colonies were slightly larger after inoculation on to pre-reduced media.

With selective media the results were variable. Quantitative recovery of some fusobacteria was better on media without Tween, but equally good on NEG and NAL. *F. mortiferum* produced larger colonies on NAL. Pigmented bacteroides grew equally well on all three media, but pigmentation developed more quickly on media containing Tween (NAT). Anaerobic cocci in general grew better on Wilkins-Chalgren agar, and produced larger colonies with Tween (NAT). Peptostreptococci, however, showed no preference. The quantitative recovery of most clostridia was much reduced on any media containing nalidixic acid.

CONCLUSION

(1) NEG was the most suitable selective medium, and also enabled haemolytic streptococci to be recognised in mixed cultures with enterobacteria.

(2) It was not necessary to pre-reduce media before inoculation provided that plates were freshly poured.

(3) A well-controlled anaerobic jar system was at least as good as an anaerobic cabinet.

ABSTRACT 19

THE POSSIBLE ROLE OF ANAEROBES IN METHYLMALONIC ACIDURIA

AN INHERITED METABOLIC DISEASE.

S.P. Borriello, P.J. Reed, M. Bain, M. Jones, M. Tracey, T.E. Stacey, and R.A. Chalmers

Division of Communicable Diseases and of Perinatal and Child Health, Clinical Research Centre, Watford Road, Middlesex, HA1 3UJ, UK.

Several inherited metabolic diseases (organic acidurias) are associated with defects in the metabolism of amino acids, leading to the accumulation of toxic, fatty-acyl CoA esters and their metabolites in tissues and body fluids, These metabolites can be associated with severe life-threatening episodes. Treatment includes dietary protein restriction and the use of vitamin co-factors at pharmacological doses.

Methylmalonic aciduria (MMA) is an inherited disorder of isoleucine and valine metabolism in which accumulation of methylmalonyl CoA and its metabolic precursor propionyl CoA in urine and body fluids are associated with develop-mental problems as well as being life-threatening. The possible role of the gut flora in contributing to the metabolite load in this and similar diseases has rarely been considered.

We have shown that a patient with MMA improved clini-cally and biochemically during treatment with amoxycillin and with metronidazole. During the latter course, urinary methylmalonic acid (MM) and propionic acid, which can be converted to MM, were estimated over a period of 40 days before and 90 days during metronidazole treatment (11 mg/kg/day). Urinary MM fell from 12.8 mole/mole creatinine (SD 4.21, n = 17) to 3.5 (SD 1.5, n = 15), P <0.001, and stool propionate fell from 101 micromole/ml stool (SD 5.3, n = 13), to 2.1 (SD 6.8, n = 23), P <0.001.

The levels of faecal propionate before metronidazole therapy were greatly elevated compared to healthy subjects whose levels in three age matched controls and three adults were 17.2 and 16.4 micromoles/gm respectively. Interestingly, both during and after metronidazole therapy, the total numbers of bacteria capable of producing propionate *in vitro* remained at 10^9/gm of stool, which is the same as for healthy adults. The overall effects on the faecal flora are presented in the table. The most significant effect was the removal of clostridia, bacteroides and veillonella.

Table.

Micro-organism	3 mths into metronidazole treatment	1 day post metronidazole treatment	2 wks post metronidazole treatment
Total facultatives	8×10^9	2×10^{10}	10^{10}
Total strict AnO$_2$	–	–	3×10^{10}
Staphylococci	8×10^9	2×10^{10}	10^8
Bacilli	10^4*	$6 \times 10^{3*}$	10^{10*}
Proteus	10^7	10^7	10^9
Coliforms	–	2×10^9	–
Yeasts	1.5×10^4	8×10^5	–
Clostridia	–	–	6×10^6 $(4 \times 10^{3*})$
Bacteroides	–	–	3×10^{10} $(2 \times 10^{9*})$
Veillonella	–	–	$1.4 \times 10^{8*}$
Propionic acid producing potential	10^7	10^9	10^9

*No./gm of stool producing propionate *in vitro*
-None detected

It appears that propionic acid production by the faecal flora was suppressed by metronidazole, even though the total numbers of bacteria capable of producing propionic acid were not decreased. Interestingly, in addition to its effect on the anaerobic flora there was some evidence that a propionic acid-producing facultative bacillus was affected.

The findings suggest a previously largely unexplored metabolic role for the intestinal flora in contributing to the accumulation of fatty products that occur in organic

ABSTRACT 20

INFLUENCE OF SULPHATASE-PRODUCING INTESTINAL BACTERIA ON THE METABOLISM OF BILE SALTS AND STEROID HORMONES

H. Eyssen, J. van Eldere and J. Robben.

Rega Institute, University of Leuven, Minderbroedersstraat 10, B-3000 Leuven, Belgium.

Sulphation of bile salts and steroid hormones promotes the faecal excretion of these compounds and sulphatase-producing intestinal bacteria might interfere with these processes. By using strictly anaerobic techniques, we isolated seven sulphatase-producing bacteria from the human and rat intestinal flora. Substrate specificity was studied *in vitro*; the *in vivo* effects were studied in gnotobiotic rats associated with these strains.

Strains S-1 and S-2 were fastidious and asaccharolytic *Clostridium* species isolated from rats. Strain S-1 desulphated the 3 α -sulphates of the normal 5 β -bile salts, but not the 3 α -sulphates of the 5α - or allo-bile salts. In gnotobiotic rats, *Clostridium* S-1 prolonged the half-life of labelled cholate-3-sulphate from 2.7 days in germfree rats to 12.2 days in gnotobiotic rats associated with this strain. The fraction of faecal cholate presenting as the 3-sulphate ester decreased from 26% in germfree to 0% in the S-1 associated rats. S-1 had no effect on the sulphation of faecal allochenodeoxycholate. Strain S-2 desulphated both types of bile salts and in gnotobiotic rats associated with S-2 faecal excretion of allochenodeoxycholate decreased from 10% in germfree rats to less than

1% in the gnotobiotic animals, due to desulphation and subsequent transformation to isoallocheno- deoxycholate by S-2. Strains S-1 and S-2 also desulphated certain arylsulphates, e.g. estrone-3-sulphate, but were inactive on alkylsulphates, e.g. cholestane, pregnane or androstane sulphates.

Table. Substrate specificity.

3-Sulphate esters of	Rat strains			Human strains			
	S-1	S-2	R-9	H-1	H-2	H-3	H-4
Bile salts							
3α OH-5β bile salts	+	+	−	−	−	o	o
3α OH-5β bile salts	+	−	−	−	−	o	o
3α OH-5β bile salts	−	+	−	−	−	o	o
Aryl							
estrone	+	+	+	+	+	+	+
17β-estradiol	+	+	+	+	+	+	+
estriol	−	−	−	o	o	o	o
p-nitrocatechol	+	+	−	o	o	o	o
p-nitrophenol	+	+	−	o	o	o	o
Alkyl							
dehydroisoandrosterone	−	−	−	−	−	−	+
5α-androstane-3β-ol-17-one	−	−	−	−	−	o	o
5α-androstane-3α-ol-17-one	−	−	−	−	−	o	o
5α-pregnane-3β-ol-20-one	−	−	−	−	−	o	o
cholesterol	−	−	−	−	−	o	o
coprostanol	−	−	−	−	−	o	o

+ : positive;   − : negative;   o : not tested.

Strain R-9, a Gram-positive unidentified anaerobic rod isolated from rat caecum, was inactive on bile salt sulphates but desulphated estrone-3- sulphate; the substrate specificity for non-steroid arylsulphates was, however, different from strain S-1 and S-2. Strain R-9 was also inactive on alkylsulphates. Association of germfree rats with strains S-1 or R-9 showed a small but significant decrease of the faecal excretion of intraperitoneally injected labelled estrone-3-sulphate. From human faecal material, we isolated four sulphatase-acidurias.

producing strains termed H-1, H-2, H-3 and H-4. Strains H-1 and H-2 were inactive on bile salt sulphates and alkyl-sulphates such as pregnane and androstane sulphates, but they desulphated estrone-3-sulphate. H-1 and H-2 were closely related to *Eubacterium cylindroides*.

Strain H-4 differed from all other strains in its ability to desulphate dehydroisoandrosterone-3-sulphate, an alkylsulphate.

ABSTRACT 21

FOOD ADDITIVE METABOLISM BY INTESTINAL BACTERIA IN MAN

P. Geraldine S. Cook.

London School of Hygiene and Tropical Medicine, Keppel Street, London, WC1E 7HT, UK.

The effect of food additives upon the faecal floras was found to result in changes in enzyme activities when compared with a control period. Investigations have centred upon the coal tar dye tartrazine (E102) (2). Changes in azoreductase activity and of the collection of nineteen enzymes detected in the A.P.I. ZYM strip were studied. The protocol used throughout the study was an initial seven days of control dietary period, followed by seven days of the control diet plus the additives under test. This protocol was a single crossover, monitored over fourteen days. The work shows that the intake of dietary tartrazine, at the level comparable to a normal human dose (A.D.I. levels), does produce detectable enzymatic alterations to bacterial organisms. Bile acid changes were additionally detected in this study, as has been noted by others (1).

References

1   Allen, R.J. and Roxon J.J. 1974. Metabolism by
     intestinal bacterial organisms and the effect of bile
     acids upon tartrazine azoreduction.
     Xenobiotica 4(10),637-643.

2   Commision of the European Community. 1980. Food
     Additives and the Consumer. Luxenbourg

ABSTRACT 22

MAINTENANCE IN CONTINUOUS CULTURE OF THE GASTRIC MICROFLORA OF A HYPOCHLORHYDRIC PATIENT

T.M. Coutts*, A.J. Alldrick*, I.R. Rowland*,
J.M. Dolby and S.P. Borriello

*BIBRA, Carshalton, Surrey.   CRC, Watford Road, Middlesex.

Hypochlorhydria (reduced secretion of gastric acid) is a clinical condition common in the elderly and frequently associated with diseases such as pernicious anaemia and hypogammaglobulinaemia. It is characterised by elevated gastric pH and bacterial colonisation of the normally sterile stomach (1,2). These altered conditions may favour bacterial transformation of ingested chemicals leading to potentially toxic or clinical sequelae, reactions of particular interest being the reduction of nitrate to nitrite and the nitrosation of amines to form mutagenic and carcinogenic nitrosamines. To study the reactions catalysed by the hypochlorhydric stomach microflora presents difficulties both in vivo and in vitro.

Continuous culture has been used successfully to model the hind gut microflora of the rat and human and so may provide a suitable method for modelling the mixed bacterial flora of the hypochlorhydric stomach and thus facilitate metabolic studies.

A mixture of organisms isolated from the gastric

juice of a patient with hypogammaglobulinaemia was used to inoculate a medium based on brain heart infusion and yeast extract and cultured under continuous flow conditions. The culture, dilution rate 0.08 per hr, was maintained at 37°C and at pH 8.0 which was the pH of the gastric juice obtained from the patient. Under these conditions a mixed population of all the strains in the original inoculum, consisting of four strains of streptococci, two strains of staphylococci and a veillonella was maintained at a cell density of 1 - 1.6 x 10^9 viable cells/ml for 13 weeks.

The culture expressed a range of enzyme activities as judged by a semi-quantitative assay method (API ZYM) and in addition was capable of reducing nitrate to nitrite and of hydrolysing glycosides. The activities of nitrate reductase (mean activity 0.11 micromole nitrite produced per ml/hr) and beta-glycosidase (mean activity 0.72 micromole glycoside hydolysed/ml/hr) varied considerably over the experimental period.

The study has demonstrated that it is possible to maintain *in vitro* a mixed bacterial population which reflects, in species diversity, the gastric flora of a patient with hypochlorhydria. The enzyme activities associated with the culture lead to the production of nitrite and glycosides both of which may have toxicological consequences for the patient.

Acknowledgements

This study had the approval of the Northwick Park Hospital Ethical Committee. We thank Dr A.D.B. Webster for samples of gastric juices. TMC, AJA and IRR were supported by funds provided by U.K. Ministry of Agriculture, Fisheries and Food.

References

1   Dolby, J.M., Webster, A.D.B., Borriello, S.P.,
     Barclay, F.E., Bartholomew, B.A. and Hill, M.J.
     1984. Bacterial colonization and nitrite
     concentration in the Aclorhydric stomachs of patients
     with primary Hypogammaglobulinaemia or classical
     Pernicious anaemia.
     Scand. J. Gasteroenterol. 19: 105-110.

2   Stockbruegger, R.W., Cotton, P.B., Menon, G.G.,
     Beilby, J.O.W., Bartholomew, B.A., Hill, M.J. and
     Walters, C.L. 1984. Pernicious Anaemia,
     Intragastric bacterial overgrowth and possible
     consequences. Scand. J. Gastroenterology 19: 355-
     364.

ABSTRACT   23

A CHEMOSTAT MODEL FOR FORMATION OF BACTERIAL FILMS ON ACRYLIC TILES.

D.J. Bradshaw, A.B. Dowsett* and C.V. Keevil

Bacterial Metabolism Research Laboratory and *Experimental
Pathology Laboratory, PHLS Centre for Applied Microbiology
& Research, Porton Down, Salisbury, Wiltshire SP4 OJG, UK.

In natural ecosystems, microbial activity and growth

is often associated with the presence of a surface,

particularly in low nutrient environments. The chemostat

allows the study of such environments by manipulation of

the nutrient limitation, together with the precise control

of other parameters, such as slow growth rates and pH.

Thus the chemostat may provide an environmentally-related

model (a microcosm) in which in vivo-like activity of a

multi-component system can be simulated. Enrichment

cultures of bacterial communities can be obtained in the

chemostat and it is apparent that growth is enhanced on a

surface compared to that in the surrounding medium (1).

Of particular interest is the attachment of oral bacteria

to tooth enamel, prior to the formation of plaque, with

resultant malodour due to bacterial metabolism and the

potential development of a carious lesion. We have investigated this attachment process by modifying a fermenter
head so that acrylic tiles can be immersed in a continuous
culture of plaque bacteria and withdrawing the tiles at
regular intervals for microbiological analysis and
scanning electron microscopy.

The fermenter head was redesigned in autoclavable
nylon with the usual number of ports, for housing elect-
rodes etc. An additional eight ports around the periphery
allowed the insertion and retrieval of tiles which were
autoclaved and introduced aseptically during continuous
culture. Plaque was collected aseptically from the teeth
of 13 schoolchildren and was taken to the laboratory in
anaerobic transport medium to be pooled and stored in
liquid nitrogen. Aliquots were inoculated into complex
medium (2) and the community established at pH 7.0 and a
dilution rate of $0.05hr^{-1}$.

Good growth of streptococci, veillonella, fusobacteria
and neisseria was obtained with reduced numbers of lactobacilli and actinomyces when the glucose concentration was
limiting (28mM). *Bacteroides* spp. only established when
the medium was supplemented with haemin and vitamin K.
Analysis of the tiles indicated that bacteria growing in
the culture invariably attached to the immersed surfaces
in a reproducible manner. Scanning electron microscopy
confirmed that fusiforms attached to both smooth and, in
particular, rough surfaces of the tiles before cocci and
grew as large sheets. Cocci attached later on to the
remaining smooth surfaces. The climax community established within 14 days when corn-cob formation was evident.

References

1   Ellwood, D.C., Keevil, C.W., Marsh, P.D., Brown, C.M.
     and Wardell, J.N. 1982.   Surface-associated growth.
     Phil. Trans. R. Soc. Lond. B. 297: 517-532.

2   Shah,H.N., Williams, R.A.D., Bowden, G.H. and Hardie,
     J.M. 1976. Comparison of the biochemical properties
     of *Bacteroides melaninogenicus* from human dental
     plaque and other sites.
     J. Appl. Bacteriol. 41: 473-492.

ABSTRACT   24

CHARACTERISATION OF COLONIAL VARIANTS OF *BACTEROIDES*

GINGIVALIS W50 WITH AN ALTERED VIRULENCE FOR MICE

Ailsa S. McKee, Ann S. McDermid, A.B. Dowsett,
     A. Baskerville and P.D. Marsh.

PHLS, Centre for Applied Microbiological Research, Porton
Down, Salisbury, Wiltshire. SP4 0JG, UK.

Bacteroides   gingivalis is   an   asaccharolytic,

obligately   anaerobic   Gram-negative   rod   implicated   in

advanced   periodontitis in man (4,2).   This organism   when

grown in either batch or continuous culture has been shown

to be pathogenic in mice when the essential growth   factor

haemin is in excess in the culture medium (5, 1).

In   this study colonial variants were observed   when

small volumes of chemostat culture were plated on to blood

agar plates.   In addition to the predominant typical black

pigmenting   colonies,   "biege"   and   brown   colonies   were

observed   after   10-14 days   anaerobic   incubation.   These

different   colony   types remained pure on   subculture   but

when   incubated for periods in excess of 21 days did   show

some   degree   of pigmentation.   Different colonial   types

were   grown in a chemostat in a complex   medium,   BM   (3),

under   haemin limitation, < 0.5mcg/ml haemin,   or   haemin excess, $>= 0.5mcg/ml$, at a dilution rate $D = 0.1h^{-1}$ (MGT = 6.9h), pH 7.5   0.2 and 37°C.   In contrast to the original black-pigmenting colony culture growth,   which was pathogenic in mice under high haemin concentrations ($>0.5mcg/ml$) but   showed   reduced   virulence when haemin   was   limiting growth,   the   "biege"   colony chemostat   culture   was   not pathogenic   in   mice   irrespective of the   haemin   concentration.   Acid   end-product analysis of both the   "biege" and   black colony growth in BM indicated that   the   acidic products of metabolism were acetic, propionic, isobutyric, butyric,   iso-valeric and phenylacetic acids, the presence of   the latter acid being one of the significant   criteria used in distinguishing *B.gingivalis* from *B.asaccharolyticus* (4) which is non pathogenic in mice.   Preliminary investigation   of   outer membrane protein pattern profiles   using SDS polyacrylamide gel electrophoresis indicated that   the "biege" and black colony growth gave very similar patterns with   a few reproducible differences.   Gluteraldehyde   and ruthenium   red   treated cells were sectioned and   examined under the electron microscope.   Differences were observed in the staining of the extracellular material produced   by the   two colonial variants.   Further study of this extracellular   material may assist in the understanding of   the virulence of this organism.

References

1   McKee, A.S., McDermid, A.S., Marsh, P.D. and Ellwood, D.C. 1984. The application of continuous culture techniques to the study of oral anaerobes. p165-175. In: M.J. Hill (ed.) Models of Anaerobic Infection. Martinus Nijhoff Publishers, Bordrect.

2   Moore, W.E.C., Holdeman, L.V., Smibert, R.M., Hash, D.E., Burmeister, J.A. and Ranney, R.R. 1982. Bacteriology of severe periodontitis in young adult humans. Infect. Immun. 38: 1137-1148.

3   Shah, H.N., Williams, R.A.D., Bowden, G.H. and
     Hardie, J.M. 1976. Comparison of the biochemical
     properties of *Bacteroides melaninogenicus* from human
     dental plaque and other sites.
     J. Appl. Bacteriol. 41: 473-492.

4   Slotts, J. 1982. Importance of black-pigmented
     bacteroides in human periodontal disease. p27-45. In:
     R.J. Genco and S.E. Mergenhagen (eds.) Host-parasite
     interactions in periodontal diseases. American
     Society for Microbiology. Washington D.C.

5   van Steenbergen, T.J.M., Kastelein, P., Touw, J.J.A.
     and de Graaff, J. 1982. Virulence of black-
     pigmented bacteroides strains from periodontal
     pockets and other sites in experimentally induced
     skin lesions in mice. J. Periodont. Res. 17: 41-49.

ABSTRACT   25

THE GROWTH OF *ACTINOMYCES NAESLUNDII* IN THE DENTAL PLAQUE
OF MONKEYS (MACACA FASCICULARIS)

D. Beighton and H.Hayday.

Royal College of Surgeons of England, Dental Research
Unit, Downe, Kent, U.K.

Microaerophilic actinomyces (*Actinomyces naeslundii*
and *A.viscosus*) are ubiquitous in the dental plague of
animals (4). We have previously reported the acquisition
of actinomyces in monkeys and the influence of dietary
composition on their proportions in plaque (1).   Here we
have used a model for determining the number of bacteria
in developmental grooves on teeth (3) to estimate the
growth rate of actinomyces and to determine the influence
of diet withdrawal on their growth.

Monkeys (20-28 months old) were fed a low sucrose
maintenance diet.   Plaque of known age (0-96 h) was
removed from each monkey, dispersed and the total number
of bacteria and the number of actinomyces per groove
determined.   Total counts were made on HBA plus menadione

and incubated anaerobically. Actinomyces were cultured on supplemented BHIA, with NaF and colistin (2) and incubated in 10% (v/v) carbon dioxide and identified as previously described (1). Bacterial counts were transformed to $\log_{10}$ prior to analysis.

A. naeslundii was the predominant actinomyces isolated. Their number per groove increased from 0.38×10^2 to 0.61×10^4 between 6 and 24 hr. and remained relatively constant up to 96 hr. Similarly, the total number of bacteria increased from 0.32×10^4 at 0 h to 0.23×10^6 at 18h. Doubling time of *A. naeslundii* during the 6 to 24 hr period was (mean +/- sd) 3.25 +/- 2.89 hr (median = 2.72; range 1.24-11.66 hr) and for the total number of bacteria 3.57 ± 1.93 (median 2.91 hr; range 1.75-9.03h.). These data

Table 1. The effect of food withdrawal, with or without water supplementation with 1 per cent (w/v) glucose, for 18hr on the number (mean $\log_{10}$ +/- sd) of bacteria and *Actinomyces naeslundii* per groove (n = 12).

Bacteria	Fed by mouth + water	Dietary regimen Food withdrawn + water	Food withdrawn + 1% glucose in water
Total cfu (anaerobic)	6.29 ± 0.24	6.27 ± 0.33	6.28 ± 0.45
Total actinomyces	4.53 ± 0.52	4.64 ± 0.88	4.58 ± 0.50
A. naeslundii	4.41 ± 0.54	4.56 ± 0.90	4.34 ± 0.73
Total streptococci	5.40 ± 0.52	5.60 ± 0.56	5.69 ± 0.63

demonstrate that *A. naeslundii* grows at a relatively rapid rate in immature dental plaque.

The ability of *A. naeslundii* to grow on saliva was studied by fasting monkeys for 18h and providing them with distilled water or distilled water with 1% glucose. There were no significant differences between the total number of bacteria or the number of *A. naeslundii* per groove when the monkeys were fed or fasted (table).

The failure to change the numbers of *A. naeslundii* per groove by the withdrawal of the diet indicates that *A.naeslundii* is able to obtain its nutritional require- ments from saliva alone. Further, the factors limiting the rate of growth of *A. naeslundii* in developing plaque may not be the lack of carbohydrate or any other specific nutritional requirement but rather the growth rate may be controlled by the antibacterial systems of saliva.

References

1   Beighton, D. 1985. Establishment and distribution of
    the bacteria *Actinomyces viscosus* and *Actinomyces
    naeslundii* in the mouths of monkeys (*Macaca
    fascicularis*). Archs oral Biol. 30: 403-407.

2   Beighton, D. and Colman, G. 1976. A medium for the
    isolation and enumeration of oral *Actinomycetaceae*
    from dental plaque. J. Dent. Res. 55: 875-878.

3   Beighton, D., Hayday, H. and Walker, J. 1985. The
    relationship between the number of the bacterium
    Streptococcus mutans at discrete sites on the
    dentition of macaque monkeys (*Macaca fascicularis*)
    and the subsequent development of dental caries.
    Archs oral Biol. 30: 85-88.

4   Dent, V.E. and Marsh, P.D. 1981. Evidence for a
    basic plaque microbial community on the tooth surface
    in animals. Archs oral Biol. 26: 171-179.

ABSTRACT   26

ATTACHING SPIROCHAETES IN THE PIG COLON

R.J. Lysons, A.P. Bland and M.R. Burrows.

Institute for Research on Animal Diseases, Compton, Berkshire, UK.

Spirochaetes attaching to colonic epithelial cells have been reported in a number of animal species. A similar phenomenon was observed in seven pigs which were seven to ten weeks of age. The bacteria formed a very dense layer which could be recognised by light microscopy as a basophilic haze on the epithelial surface. Scanning electron microscopy confirmed that these were spirochaetes. Using a morphometric point counting technique (1), 63% of the colonic surface of one specimen was shown to be covered in spirochaetes.

Attaching spirochaetes have been implicated in a porcine colonic disease syndrome by Taylor *et al.* (2). Investigations were carried out on pigs from 4 herds which had a similar colonic disease but in this study there was not a good association between these spirochaetes and disease. The pigs with attaching spirochaetes had all

Table. Attempts to transmit diarrhoeal disease by exposure of susceptible pigs to colonic tissue from affected pigs

Exp. no.		No. of pigs	No. with lesions
I	Exposed	6	4
	Controls	6	0
II	Exposed	6	4
	Controls	6	0

suffered episodes of diarrhoea caused by colitis; these, however, only represented a small proportion of animals with the disease. When examined by transmission electron microscopy the epithelial cells to which the bacteria were attached appeared morphologically normal.

To assess whether this diarrhoeal syndrome was trans-missible, chopped pieces of colon wall from four affected pigs were fed to six pigs from herds which had not experienced this problem (table).

In both experiments the pigs were exposed to colonic tissue on which attaching spirochaetes were detected. However, in none of the eight pigs which developed lesions (table) could attaching spirochaetes be demonstrated.

The above evidence suggests that the porcine diarrhoeal syndrome examined in this study is transmissible, but that the attaching spirochaete is not the causal organism.

References

1   Ried, I.M. 1980. Morphometrics in veterinary pathology - a review. Vet. Path. 17: 522-543.

2   Taylor, D.J., Simmons, J.R. and Laird, H.M. 1980. Production of diarrhoea and dysentery in pigs by feeding pure cultures of a spirochaete differing from *Treponema hyodysenteriae*. Vet. Rec. 196: 324-330.

ABSTRACT 27

PLASMIDS IN STEROID NUCLEAR DEHYDROGENATING CLOSTRIDIA

Daphne E. Thompson, B.S. Drasar* and A.R. Cook

Bacterial Metabolism Research Laboratory, PHLS, Centre for Applied Microbiology and Research, Porton Down, Salisbury, Wiltshire, UK.

* London School of Hygiene and Tropical Medicine, Keppel Street, London, UK.

Intestinal clostridia which dehydrogenate the steroid nucleus (nuclear dehydrogenating clostridia, NDC) are implicated in the aetiology of colorectal cancer. Hill (1) proposed that these clostridia could metabolise bile acids to compounds, such as 3oxo-chola,1,4,dienoic acid, which are structurally similar to known carcinogens.

NDC are the only intestinal bacteria known to be

capable of this nuclear dehydrogenation *in vitro*. The reaction has not been directly demonstrated *in vivo* but trace amounts of 3-oxo-4-cholenic acid have been detected in faeces. Indirect evidence is provided by the presence of allo bile acids in faeces (5) which are produced via a 4-ene intermediate.

The 3oxo-steroid nuclear dehydrogenase is not associated with a single clostridial species suggesting that it may be extra- chromosomally encoded. Natural transfer of such an element to clostridia previously lacking the enzyme activity could alter levels of potential carcinogens present in the gut thus modulating colorectal cancer risk.

In a previous study (2) 93% of *Clostridium paraputrificum* 90% of *C. tertium* and below 31% of some other clostridial species were NDC positive. These three groups of NDC were analysed for plasmid content using an alkaline extraction method (Table).

Table. Plasmid isolation from NDC positive strains.

	Clostridium species	Molecular Weight (Md)								
D2	*C. paraputrificum*	3.16	6.16	8.3	30.9					
D53	*C. paraputrificum*	2.75	3.16	5.0	5.56	6.7	7.6	8.3	16.2	30.9
D58	*C. paraputrificum*	2.34	2.75	3.0	3.63	4.36	5.0	6.02	8.3	12.3
D67	*C. paraputrificum*	2.75	3.16	5.0	5.56	6.7	7.6	14.1	17.1	
D68ii	*C. paraputrificum*	3.16	5.0	5.56	6.7	7.6	8.3	16.2	30.9	
D69i	*C. paraputrificum*	2.75	3.16	5.0	5.56	6.7	7.6	8.3	16.2	30.9
D78	*C. fallax*	3.31	5.12	7.4	15.5					
D63	*C. innocuum*	None isolated								
D19	*C. fallax*	5.12	15.5							
D49	*C. celatum*	3.31	6.3							
D46	*C. fallax*	2.88	3.55	5.12	8.7	17.3				
D119i	*C. butyricum*	None isolated								
D18	*C. sp.*	None isolated								
D45	*C. clostridiiformis*	3.31								
D117	*C. chauvoei*	4.7	6.45	12.6	25.7					
D18	*C. sartagoformum*	None isolated								
D59i	*C. butyricum*	2.88	5.5	8.3	11.2	18.6	35.4			
D119ii	*C. sartagoformum*	None isolated								
T3	*C. tertium*	5.75								
T4	*C. tertium*	17.7								
T8	*C. tertium*	5.75	17.7							
T21	*C. tertium*	5.75	17.7							
T17	*C. tertium*	None isolated								
T16	*C. tertium*	None isolated								

Plasmids were isolated from all NDC positive strains of *C. paraputrificum* and from some strains of *C. tertium* and the less common species of NDC. We did not isolate any large plasmids, which would be necessary to effect plasmid transfer. This may be related to the high intracellular endonuclease activity associated with clostridia (4). Curing with flavin dyes and elevated temperatures resulted in permanent loss of both plasmids and enzyme activity for three consecutive subcultures, but of 1460 colonies tested no stable NDC negative clones were obtained. Curing rates reported for clostridia are low 0.3% (3) therefore further work is required before it can be concluded that the enzyme is not extrachromosomally encoded.

Acknowledgement

Daphne Thompson gratefully acknowledges the Cancer Research Campaign, U.K. for financing this work.

References

1   Hill, M.J. 1977. The Role of Unsaturated Bile Acids in the Etiology of Large Bowel Cancer. In: Hiatt, H.H. (ed.) The Origins of Human Cancer. Cold Spring Harbour. p1634.

2   Hill, M.J. 1985. Clostridia and Human Colorectal Cancer. In: S.P. Borriello (ed.) Clostridia in Gastrointestinal Disease. CRC Press, Boca Raton, Florida. p171.

3   Rood, J.I. Scott, V.N. and Duncan, C.L. 1978. Identification of transferable tetracycline resistance plasmid (PCW3) from *Clostridium perfringens*. Plasmid 1: 563-570.

4   Urano, N., Karube, I., Suzuki, S., Yamada, T., Hirochika, H. and Sakaguchi, K. 1983. Isolation and partial characterisation of large plasmids in hydrogen-evolving bacterium, *Clostridium butyricum*. Eur. J. Appl. Microbiol. Biotechnol. 17: 349-354.

5   Wait, R. and Thompson, M.H. 1984. Minor faecal bile acids and large bowel cancer. Biochem. Soc. Trans. 12: 1134.